CLEAR BODY CLEAR MIND

THE EFFECTIVE PURIFICATION PROGRAM

L. RON HUBBARD

CLEAR BODY CLEAR MIND

THE EFFECTIVE PURIFICATION PROGRAM

Bridge

PUBLICATIONS, INC.

A HUBBARD PUBLICATION

Published in the U.S.A. by
Bridge Publications, Inc.
4751 Fountain Avenue
Los Angeles, California 90029

ISBN 0-88404-549-8

Published in all other countries by
NEW ERA Publications International, ApS
Store Kongensgade 55
1264 Copenhagen K, Denmark

ISBN 87-7336-734-6

This book is part of the works of L. Ron Hubbard, who developed *Scientology* ®
applied religious philosophy. It is presented to the reader as a record of
observations and research into the nature of the human mind and spirit, and
not as a statement of claims made by the author. The benefits and goals of
Scientology can be attained only by the dedicated efforts of the reader.

The *Purification* program cannot be construed as a recommendation of medical
treatment or medication and it is not professed as a physical handling for
bodies nor is any claim made to that effect. There are no medical
recommendations or claims for the *Purification* program or for any of the
vitamin or mineral regimens described in this book.

No individual should undertake the *Purification* program or any of its regimens
without first consulting and obtaining the informed approval of a licensed
medical practitioner. The author makes no warranties or representation as to
the effectiveness of the *Purification* program.

Purification, Purification Rundown and *Purif* are trademarks for the
detoxification program described in this book and are used as such in the
writings of L. Ron Hubbard. They are registered as service marks and are
owned by Religious Technology Center. These marks may not be used as
designations for the detoxification program given in this work without the
prior consent of Religious Technology Center.

Hubbard and *Scientology* are trademarks and service marks owned by Religious
Technology Center.

Printed in the United States of America

Important Note

In reading this book, be very certain you never go past a word you do not fully understand.

The only reason a person gives up a study or becomes confused or unable to learn is because he or she has gone past a word that was not understood.

The confusion or inability to grasp or learn comes AFTER a word that the person did not have defined and understood.

Have you ever had the experience of coming to the end of a page and realizing you didn't know what you had read? Well, somewhere earlier on that page you went past a word that you had no definition for or an incorrect definition for.

Here's an example. "It was found that when the crepuscule arrived the children were quieter and when it was not present, they were much livelier." You see what happens. You think you don't understand the whole idea, but the inability to understand came entirely from the one word you could not define, *crepuscule,* which means twilight or darkness.

It may not only be the new and unusual words that you will have to look up. Some commonly used words can often be misdefined and so cause confusion.

This datum about not going past an undefined word is the most important fact in the whole subject of study. Every subject you have taken up and abandoned had its words which you failed to get defined.

Therefore, in studying this book be very, very certain you never go past a word you do not fully understand. If the material becomes confusing or you can't seem to grasp it, there will be a word just earlier that you have not understood. Don't go any further, but go back to BEFORE you got into trouble, find the misunderstood word and get it defined.

Definitions

As an aid to the reader, words most likely to be misunderstood have been defined in footnotes the first time they occur in the text. Words sometimes have several meanings. The footnote definitions in this book only give the meaning that the word has as it is used in the text. Other definitions for the word can be found in a dictionary.

A glossary including all the footnote definitions is at the back of this book.

Foreword

by John Duff, co-author of
The Truth About Drugs

We live in a society under siege, bombarded by an onslaught of drugs and toxins. There is no part of life on this planet today that is not being destroyed by this assault—from the upper strata of society to the children of the ghettos, from the industrialized superpowers to the Brazilian rain forests. Headlines cry out the toll of individuals, families, schools, nations and entire civilizations being eaten away by poisonous drugs, chemicals and environmental toxins.

The statistics on drug abuse alone are staggering. The production, distribution and consumption of illegal drugs has become the largest and most destructive industry on Earth. Current estimates of the size of the industry vary between five hundred billion and one trillion dollars annually. The US Chamber of Commerce estimates that drug and alcohol abuse in America alone costs business some 177 billion dollars a year in drug testing, drug education for employees and lost productivity.

Drug abuse now begins in elementary school. The percentage of American grade school students who use drugs has tripled over the last decade. Today the average age that a child finds out about drugs in North America is eight years old. Almost before he can add and subtract, he learns about marijuana, LSD, cocaine and other drugs from his peers. By the time he is twelve, he must make the decision whether or not he will use drugs, as he will almost certainly be offered them right on his own school grounds.

By senior year in high school, seven out of ten students will have said "yes" to drugs. Eighty percent of the population have used illegal drugs by their mid-twenties.

While marijuana was the "street drug of choice" of the 1960s and 1970s, cocaine and its highly addictive cousin crack are now rampant in American cities. Every day, five thousand Americans try cocaine for the first time. Thousands of babies are born each year to crack-addicted mothers.

No country is immune from the ravages of drugs. Even in the Eastern bloc, drug abuse is a recognized epidemic. An article entitled "Drugs Mean Death" in Pravda, the official newspaper of the Communist Party, points out that drug abuse is a serious problem in the Soviet Union.

Along with a more pervasive, more murderous drug trade there are new stronger drugs. The so-called designer drugs are chemically designed to produce strong mind-altering effects and yet still be technically within the confines of biochemical law. Some of these designer drugs are millions of times more potent than heroin. A pinhead quantity of one has the capability of killing fifty people.

Related to the escalation of drug use is the epidemic of crime. According to the US Justice Department, America has suffered a 43 percent increase in violent crime during the past ten years, coincident with the rise in drug use. With drug habits costing between one hundred fifty and one thousand dollars per day, over 80 percent of addicts turn to crime. In New York City, 86 percent of those arrested for crime test positive for drug use.

Not everyone is the victim of a drug-related crime or knows someone who is on drugs. But drug and alcohol abuse affects everyone.

The drug our children most often first learn about from their parents is alcohol. In studies of heroin addicts, alcohol is the drug they report gave them their first "buzz." Alcohol use is heavily fortified with advertising, aimed more and more frequently at the young.

A majority of teenagers routinely drink at parties and only 8 percent report no alcohol use. Over one third of American alcoholics (3.3 million out of 9 million total) are under the legal drinking age.

The abuse of medical drugs is yet another problem. There is a dichotomy between "medical" and "recreational" drug use, with "recreational" use as the target for correction. Yet this dichotomy ignores the fact that "recreational drugs" have started out under the "medical" category. Cocaine is used for nose operations, marijuana is considered a cure for glaucoma, morphine is a painkiller. There is in fact a crossover that blurs the distinction.

Today people with emotional problems are automatically given a drug—a symptom of how far our society has descended. Once the drug has worn off, the emotional upset remains, often along with the side effects of the drug itself.

Chemical straitjackets don't solve the problem. Abuse of medical drugs may even aggravate it. Pain pills, tranquilizers and other medical drugs prescribed by psychiatrists and doctors are poisons that can be abused, just like other drugs. They can even explode without warning—as when a woman on the psychiatric drug Anafranil opened fire on a second-grade classroom, killing one child and seriously injuring five others.

And what about the long-term effects of drug use? Here the poisoning is even more insidious. Let's examine a successful computer executive, in his late thirties. Like many in the Woodstock generation, he used drugs in college, but hasn't touched anything stronger than alcohol in ten or twelve years. Diet and health magazines have convinced him that working out at the health club is a better use of his Friday and Saturday nights.

Other than the drain on his pocketbook through tax dollars, the "drug problem" doesn't really affect him. Or does it?

Sometimes he has trouble concentrating. After a ten-hour day, to actually get through reading trade journals at night is a herculean task; he only has energy for videos. Sometimes his memory is less sharp than he'd like it to be. At his fifteenth reunion, he couldn't remember the name of his first girlfriend. He is less agile on the racquetball court.

Old age? But that doesn't account for this lessening of mental facility and a feeling that he just isn't as sharp as he remembers being in high school. In fact, if he actually thinks about it, he can probably pinpoint the slight but nevertheless quite annoying feeling that his head is made of wood. If he were to concentrate on tracing back his feelings, he might find that he started having trouble studying in college just after he was introduced to drugs. Or after an operation he had for a football injury, and the painkillers. . . .

The effects of the drugs he took may seem subtle, but they can mean the difference between excellence and mediocrity or even failure. Why? Because he no longer has the mental sharpness, energy and personal stamina to make himself an unqualified success in his field. Instead, he experiences a slight lessening of his ambitions, a compromise with his abilities and a feeling that he is a little less alive. And with these elusive barriers, he has less happiness and less success in achieving his goals.

He has, in effect, been poisoned by the drugs he took in the past which remain lodged in his system years after he is no longer taking them. And that poison works in devious ways he doesn't even realize.

The abuse of alcohol and street, medical and psychiatric drugs is actually part of a much larger problem: that of our chemically oriented society. Even if a person doesn't use drugs or alcohol, he is bombarded daily with food preservatives, atmospheric chemicals, industrial chemicals, pesticides, acid rain and toxic waste, simply by virtue of living on planet Earth.

Against these kinds of onslaughts, the individual appears defenseless. There seems to be nothing he can do to stop the bombardment of himself and his children.

These poisons are taking a terrible toll on life on our planet. The real cause for alarm is that the problem continues to escalate. Despite the drug wars and drug busts, the environmental commissions and the university studies, the problem continues to increase in magnitude.

Every day there seems to be a new discovery of another environmental menace.

Every day another child dies from crack he got at recess.

Every day an airline pilot puts the lives of thousands at risk through drugs on the job. Or a teenager threatens suicide from a combination of alcohol and pills.

And every day, the resources who could handle the problem, the brightest minds of our society, are being insidiously wasted.

Workable solutions are not being employed to combat this growing menace to our survival. The problem continues to get worse.

Until the advent of the Purification program developed by L. Ron Hubbard, there was no hope. For the first time, this book offers a real and workable solution. Take the time to read it.

John Duff, co-author with Gene Chill of the book *The Truth About Drugs,* has a Bachelor of Arts degree in Health and Human Services from California State University. He has lectured to more than 150,000 parents, students, teachers and civic organizations on the drug problem.

Contents

Introduction

by Megan Shields,
Bachelor of Science, Doctor of Medicine

Drugs, toxic chemicals, pesticides and other life-hostile elements currently pervade the society in which we live. Other than choosing to live in a sealed environment, cut off from the remainder of the race, there is no way a person can avoid exposure to these toxic influences.

The magnitude of the problem cannot be overstated. Chemical elements harmful to living tissue have been found to accumulate in the human body. This has far-reaching consequences: a person who was involved in taking drugs and who later stopped can yet be influenced by a drug, even years later. Pesticide residues found in food accumulate in the fatty tissues of the body; factory workers inhale toxic fumes from manufacturing processes; firefighters are exposed to the smoke of fires that can sometimes contain deadly poisons. Cases can be recited endlessly.

Customary medical procedures held no solution to this problem. Various "treatments" have been proffered which ranged from the psychiatric viewpoint of getting the person to believe that the problems he was experiencing from toxins were all in his mind, to the administration of drugs to suppress the symptoms exhibited. These "treatments" only serve to compound the situation.

No breakthrough was made at all until L. Ron Hubbard attacked this problem head-on.

He found that people with histories of taking drugs had less than optimum reactions to situations in life and less success in handling their jobs and relationships. When the effects of these drugs were reduced, people's ability to survive well was enhanced. Over the years Mr. Hubbard developed various methods of achieving a reduction of the effects of drugs.

In 1979 his researches, as described in this book, culminated in the Purification program. This is the first and only regimen in existence that has been shown in scientific studies to reduce the level of toxic material stored in the body, and to do so safely and without the administration of any further drugs.

L. Ron Hubbard claimed no medical results for his work; his intention was to make it possible for people to achieve future mental and spiritual improvement. However, the Purification program has extremely broad application, as all truly basic discoveries do.

In the course of my work, I have had the opportunity to observe firsthand the results of the Purification program, and have found them to be nothing less than miraculous. The people I have put through the program include patients with minor effects of residual toxins, people who were exposed to toxic chemicals on the job, casual drug users and long-term heavy drug users with bodies ravaged from the effects of those drugs. The depression, hopelessness and fear which often accompany such problems were also evident in many of these patients. Upon completion of the Purification program, these people were changed, both physically and mentally.

The common theme expressed by people who have completed the program is that they are no longer encumbered by the chemicals which were shutting off their lives. They express increased mental clarity and new hope for the future. Their lives upon completion of the program are happier, healthier and more productive.

Since the release of this program in 1979, tens of thousands of people have completed it. I have had the privilege of being able to use the program in my own practice, helping people who otherwise would have had no hope of recovery from the effects of drug and toxin residuals. In view of the increasing presence of toxic chemicals in industry, the proliferation of toxic waste and pollution and the epidemic use of destructive drugs at all levels of society, the importance of the Purification program, not only to the medical profession but to the society as a whole, becomes immediately apparent.

The Purification program developed by L. Ron Hubbard is the only procedure of its kind and it is the only detoxification program that actually works. This program is one of the major discoveries of our times. It is also one of the most vital actions that must be done to salvage a civilization that is dying from the devastating effects of drugs and toxins.

Megan Shields is a Bachelor of Science and Doctor of Medicine who practices as a medical doctor in Los Angeles, California. She has administered the delivery of L. Ron Hubbard's Purification program to over three thousand people in the course of her practice. She has also participated in independent scientific studies of the efficacy of the program.

Part 1

The Purification Program:

Theory, Principles and Elements

1

Our Biochemical Society

1

Our Biochemical Society

The planet has hit a barrier which prevents any widespread social progress—drugs and other biochemical substances.

These can put people into a condition which not only prohibits and destroys physical health but which can prevent any stable advancement in mental or spiritual well-being.

That's the situation today.

We live in a biochemical society.

Bio means "life; of living things." (It is from the Greek word *bios,* which means "life" or "way of life.")

Chemical means "of or having to do with chemicals." And chemicals are the substances, simple or complex, which are the building blocks of matter.

By *biochemical* is meant "the interaction of life forms and chemical substances."

Toxic substance is a term which has been used to describe

drugs, chemicals, or any substance shown to be poisonous or harmful to an organism. The word *toxic* comes from the Greek word *toxikon* which originally meant a poison in which arrows were dipped.

The human body is made up of certain exact chemicals and chemical compounds, and complex chemical processes go on continuously within it. Some substances, such as nutrients, air and water, are vital to the continuation of these processes and for maintaining the body's health. Some substances are relatively neutral when entered into the body, causing neither benefit nor damage. *Toxic* substances are those which upset the body's normal chemical balance or interfere with its chemical processes. Some of them can wreak havoc, blocking or perverting vital body functions and making the body ill or even killing it.

Detoxification would be the action of removing a poison or a poisonous effect from something (such as from one's body).

Toxins in Abundance

There has been an enormous volume of material written on the subject of toxic substances, their reported effects and the prospects for their handling. Examples abound in publications and news reports.

Unfortunately, the current environment is becoming permeated with these life-hostile elements. Drugs, radioactive wastes, pollutants and chemical agents of various types are all a part of the scene and, apparently, more and more prevalent as time goes on.

According to studies, even some of the things that are put in a can of peas or a can of soup are to be considered toxic.

They are preservatives and the action of a preservative is to impede decay. Yet digestion and cellular action are based on decay. In other words, those things might be great for the manufacturer as they preserve his product, *but* they could be very bad for the consumer. It is not that I am on a food faddism[1] kick[2] or a kick against preservatives; the point is that man is surrounded by toxins. This one example alone (preservatives in foods) is an example of the degree to which one can be confronted with toxic substances in the course of daily living.

And with the enemies of various countries using widespread drug addiction as a defeatist mechanism, with nations vying[3] with each other in the manufacture and testing of nuclear weapons (and so increasing the amount of radioactive material free in the environment), with painkillers and sedatives[4] so easily available and with the increased use of industrial and agricultural chemicals, to say nothing of the substances developed for chemical warfare, we face a growing problem.

Putting it quite bluntly, this society, at this time, is riddled[5] with toxic substances.

To briefly point out certain data regarding those substances which pose a threat to individuals and to society at large will bring the biochemical situation more clearly into focus.

---

1. **faddism:** the practice of following a fad (a temporary fashion, notion, manner of conduct, etc., especially one followed enthusiastically by a group), such as seeking and adhering briefly to a passing variety of unusual diets, beliefs, etc.

2. **kick:** an intense, personal, usually temporary, preference, habit or passion; a fad.

3. **vying:** competing; contending.

4. **sedatives:** drugs intended to lessen excitement, nervousness or irritation.

5. **riddled:** affected in every part; having (something) spread throughout.

11

Street Drugs[6]

Research has demonstrated that the single most destructive element present in our current culture is drugs.

The acceleration of widespread use of drugs such as LSD,[7] heroin,[8] cocaine,[9] "angel dust,"[10] marijuana[11] and a long list of others has contributed heavily to a debilitated[12] society. Reportedly, some of these can cause brain and nerve damage. Marijuana, for example, so favored by college students who are supposed to be getting bright today so they can be the executives of tomorrow, has been reported capable of causing brain atrophy.[13] Even school children have been shoved into drugs. And children of drug-taking mothers have been born as druggies.

I have even established that there is such a thing as a "drug

---

6. **street drugs:** drugs which are sold or distributed on the streets, rather than by prescription.

7. **LSD:** a crystalline solid substance which is a powerful psychedelic drug, producing temporary hallucinations and a schizophrenic psychotic state. *LSD* is an abbreviation for *l*ysergic acid *d*iethylamide.

8. **heroin:** a white, crystalline, narcotic powder, derived from morphine, formerly used as a painkiller and sedative; manufacture and importation of heroin is controlled by federal law in the US because of the danger of addiction. The word is derived from the Greek word *hero* allegedly because of the feelings of power and euphoria which it stimulates.

9. **cocaine:** a bitter, crystalline drug obtained from the dried leaves of the coca shrub; it is a local anesthetic and a dangerous, illegal stimulant.

10. **angel dust:** (*slang*) phencyclidine, an anesthetic drug used as an animal tranquilizer; also widely used in several forms as an illicit hallucinogen. Also called *PCP.*

11. **marijuana:** the dried leaves and flowers of the hemp plant, used in cigarette form as a narcotic or hallucinogen.

12. **debilitated:** reduced to *debility,* the condition of being weak or feeble; weak intellectually or morally.

13. **atrophy:** a wasting away of the body or of an organ or part, as from defective nutrition or nerve damage.

personality." It is artificial and is created by drugs. Drugs can apparently change the attitude of a person from his original personality to one secretly harboring[14] hostilities and hatreds he does not permit to show on the surface. While this may not hold true in all cases, it does establish a link between drugs and increasing difficulties with crime, production and the modern breakdown of social and industrial culture.

The devastating physiological effects of drugs are the subject of newspaper headlines routinely. That they also result in a breakdown of mental alertness and ethical fiber is all too obvious.

The drug scene is planetwide. It is swimming in blood and human misery.

But, vicious and damaging though they are, street drugs are actually only one part of the biochemical problem.

Medical and Psychiatric Drugs

Medical and most particularly psychiatric drugs (Valium,[15] Librium[16] and LSD to name but a few) can be every bit as damaging as street drugs. The prevalence of these currently in common use would be quite amazing to one unfamiliar with the problem.

---

14. **harboring:** keeping or holding in the mind; maintaining; entertaining.

15. **Valium:** trademark for a drug called diazepam, a tranquilizer that relaxes muscles and prevents or inhibits convulsions. It is addictive and is often prescribed by doctors or psychiatrists to "relieve" anxiety or tension.

16. **Librium:** trademark for a tranquilizing drug, used by psychiatrists in an attempt to suppress the symptoms of anxiety.

Phenobarbital[17] (under various brand names like Luminal and Nembutal) and other such drugs are often administered as though they were a panacea[18] for all ills. As early as 1951 many persons had become so accustomed to their daily dosage of sleeping pills or painkillers that they did not consider their little pills as drugs. More recently the drug Valium has taken its place among the tranquilizers[19] so frequently employed. But this by no means completes the list.

Too often the attitude is "If I can't find the cause of the pain, at least I'll deaden it." In the case of one mentally ill, this might read, "If he can't be made rational, at least he can be made quiet."

Unfortunately, it is not recognized that a person whose pain has been deadened by a sedative has himself been deadened by the same drug, and is much nearer the ultimate pain of death. It should be obvious that the quietest people in the world are the dead.

Commercial Processes and Products

In recent years much research has been done on the potential toxic effects of many of the substances commonly used in various commercial processes and products, and to what extent they may be finding their way into the bodies of this planet's inhabitants. Following are a few examples of what this research has brought to light.

Industrial Chemicals: Under this heading exists a vast array

---

17. **phenobarbital:** a white crystalline powder used as a sedative and hypnotic.

18. **panacea:** a supposed remedy, cure or medicine for all diseases or ills; cure-all.

19. **tranquilizers:** drugs that have a sedative or calming effect without inducing sleep.

---

of chemicals that are used in manufacturing. Not all such chemicals are toxic, of course. But workers in factories which produce or use such things as pesticides, petroleum products, plastics, detergents and cleaning chemicals, solvents, plated metals, preservatives, drugs, asbestos[20] products, fertilizers, some cosmetics, perfumes, paints, dyes, electrical equipment, or any radioactive materials can be exposed, often for extended periods, to toxic materials. And of course, the consumer can be exposed to residual amounts of such chemicals when he uses these products.

Agricultural Chemicals: Pesticides are the most obvious of the toxic substances to which workers in agricultural activities could be exposed. These include insecticides (insect-killing chemicals), man-made fertilizers and herbicides (chemicals to kill unwanted plants such as weeds).

Under the heading of herbicides come several which contain a substance known as "dioxin," known to be a highly toxic chemical, even in amounts almost too small to detect in the body. (Dioxin is found in "Agent Orange,"[21] a chemical defoliant[22] used in the Vietnam[23] War. This chemical was the

---

20. **asbestos:** any of several grayish minerals that separate into long, threadlike fibers. Because certain varieties do not burn, do not conduct heat or electricity and are often resistant to chemicals, they are used for making fireproof materials, electrical insulation, roofing, filters, etc. Known to cause lung cancer when inhaled.

21. **Agent Orange:** a powerful herbicide and defoliant containing trace amounts of dioxin, a toxic impurity suspected of causing serious health problems, including cancer and genetic damage, in some persons exposed to it, and birth defects in their offspring; used by US armed forces during the Vietnam War to defoliate jungles (1965–70). The name *Agent Orange* came from the color of the identifying stripe on the drums in which it was stored. *See also* **dioxin** and **defoliant** in the glossary.

22. **defoliant:** a chemical used to destroy or cause widespread loss of leaves, as in an area of jungle, forest, etc., used to deprive enemy troops or guerrilla forces of concealment.

23. **Vietnam:** a country in Southeast Asia; divided into North Vietnam and South Vietnam during the Vietnam War, but now reunified.

15

subject of considerable publicity when it was found that some US soldiers were exposed to it, apparently with varying adverse effects.)

Contact with chemicals used in agriculture can occur in a number of ways: The chemical can be carried on or in the plant itself and so eaten; it can be carried on the wind and be breathed in directly by those living or working in agricultural areas; or it can even be carried into drinking water supplies.

Food, Food Additives and Preservatives: There are substances added to some commercially processed foods that are meant to "enhance" color or flavor or, as mentioned above, to keep the food from spoiling. Also becoming more common are various artificial sweeteners used in "diet" soft drinks and other commercially packaged foods. From research on these "enhancers" and "preservers," it appears that a number of them are quite toxic, and the whole subject of food additives and preservatives has become a matter of concern to many people.

There is another side to this matter of food. Research findings point to the possibility that rancid[24] oils are a health hazard of a magnitude not previously suspected. Oils used in cooking or commercial processing of foods, where they are not fresh, pure and free of rancidity, have been linked by researchers with digestive and muscular ills, and even cancer.

Perfumes and Fragrances: Use of perfumes and fragrances in all sorts of products has become more and more prevalent in recent years. Everything from clothing to laundry detergent, from cellophane tape to wrapping paper is turning up with *fragrance* added to it. And that fragrance is almost always a

24. **rancid:** having a rank, unpleasant, stale smell or taste, as through decomposition, especially of fats or oils.

cheap chemical derivative, an extract of coal tar[25] which probably costs about 10 cents a fifty-gallon drum. Findings seem to bear out that these chemicals, floating about in the local supermarket as "fragrances," are actually toxic *and* can end up in the food products sold there. And when you get a mouthful of this stuff it is no aid to digestion, believe me!

Radiation: You've no doubt seen in news publications that contact with radiation can occur through exposure to nuclear weapons tests or the radioactive particles they can release into the atmosphere, nuclear wastes, or to some manufacturing processes which use radioactive materials. There are other sources of radiation exposure, too: prolonged exposure to the sun, dental and medical X-rays,[26] television sets and unshielded computer display screens are among them.

Recent research has been done into a naturally occurring radioactive gas known as radon. It is a product of the decay of another radioactive element, radium, which has been found to be present in minute amounts in the ground and in many building materials such as concrete, brick and gravel. Apparently, tiny amounts of radon gas can escape from the surfaces of such materials and thus be present in the air and inhaled. If ventilation is not provided for, the radon content of the air in a building can reportedly reach 50 to 100 times the level found outdoors.

These factors are *all* part of the biochemical problem.

---

25. **coal tar:** a thick, black, sticky liquid formed during the distillation of coal, that upon further distillation yields compounds from which are derived a large number of dyes, drugs and other synthetic compounds.

26. **X-rays:** a form of radiation similar to light but of a shorter wavelength and capable of penetrating solids; used in medicine for study, diagnosis and treatment of certain organic disorders, especially of internal structures of the body.

Any of these substances reportedly has the potential of remaining in the system.

This compounds the biochemical problem and presents a barrier of magnitude.

The most likely place for a toxic substance to lock up is in the fatty tissue. It has been said that in middle age and past middle age, a body's ability to break down fat lessens. So here we have, apparently, a situation of toxic substances locked up in fatty tissue and the fatty tissue is not actually getting broken down, and so such toxic substances could accumulate.

My interest in these somewhat brutal truths was not born only of an objective to resolve the physical ills of individuals. Rather, it was a continuation of my initial research involving the freeing of man as a spirit and handling, on this route, any barriers needing to be resolved.

The Purification program is a proffered answer to the barrier we call the biochemical problem. It could be called a "long-range detoxification program." While it is addressed primarily to the handling of drug residues lodged in the body, it is possible that there are many toxic substances which the body accumulates which the program may accelerate getting rid of.

My concern in developing the Purification program has not been with handling bodies. My research for many, many years has been carried out with the purpose of freeing man spiritually. My original inquiry was into the nature of man and the bulk of my work has always addressed man as a spiritual being. When barriers to this have arisen, those barriers have merited further research and resolution.

The Purification program was developed to meet a growing

threat to mental and spiritual advancement and well-being stemming from the more and more common use of drugs and biochemical substances in the current culture.

Its procedures do not supplant technology developed earlier, used especially in Narconon[27] drug rehabilitation centers for handling persons currently on drugs and apt to experience withdrawal symptoms[28] when taken off them. The Purification program would be begun only after such technology was applied.

There are no medicines or drugs used on the Purification program. The only dosages recommended are those classified as food. There are no medical recommendations or claims made for the program. The only claim is future spiritual improvement.

The data contained herein is a record of researches and results noted; it cannot be construed as a recommendation for medical treatment or medication, and it is undertaken or delivered by any individual on his own responsibility.

If the Purification program can be used to salvage even a part of a civilization sick from the onslaught of drugs and other toxic substances, then perhaps there is hope for all of that civilization.

---

27. **Narconon:** a drug rehabilitation program using L. Ron Hubbard's technology. It was originally organized in the Arizona State Prison by an inmate who was himself a drug addict of thirteen years. He put to use the basic principles of the mind contained in books by L. Ron Hubbard, and by doing so completely cured himself and helped twenty other inmates do the same. *Narconon* means *non-narcosis,* and there are now Narconon centers in many areas around the world. On the Narconon program, no drugs whatever are used for withdrawal, and the usual withdrawal effects, such as those experienced by quitting drugs "cold turkey," are most often completely bypassed.

28. **withdrawal symptoms:** any of various symptoms, such as profuse sweating, nausea, etc., induced in a person addicted to a drug when he is deprived of that drug.

2

The Development of the Purification Program

2

The Development of the Purification Program

What is the Purification program?

To state it simply, it is a program developed to assist in releasing and flushing out of the body the accumulated toxic residues which may be lodged in the tissues, while also rebuilding the impaired tissues and cells.

What is its genesis?[1]

Discovery that LSD Can Lodge in the System

In the 1970s, working with cases of individuals who had been drug users, and in a study of their physical symptoms and behavioral patterns, I made a startling discovery.

People who had been on LSD at some earlier time sometimes had reactions which appeared to act as if they had just taken more LSD!

As it has been stated that it takes only one millionth of an

---

1. **genesis:** the way in which something comes to be; beginning; origin.

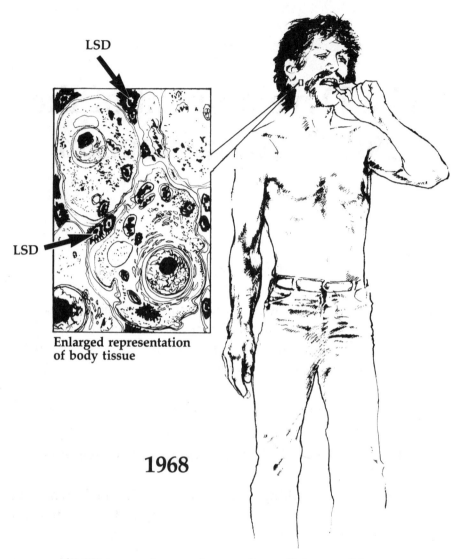

LSD

LSD

Enlarged representation
of body tissue

1968

ounce of LSD to produce a drugged condition and because it is basically wheat rust,[2] which simply cuts off circulation, my original thinking on this was that LSD must remain in the body.

---

2. **rust:** a fungus which causes any of several diseases of plants, characterized by reddish, brownish or black blisterlike swellings on the leaves, stems, etc.

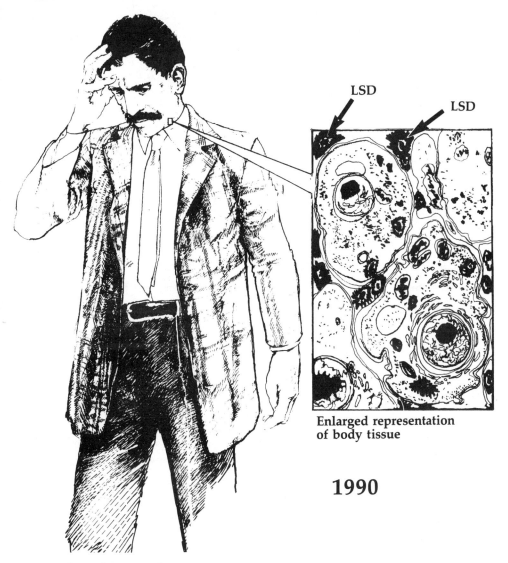

LSD

LSD

Enlarged representation of body tissue

1990

In other words:

LSD apparently stays in the system, lodging in the tissues, and mainly the fatty tissues of the body, and is liable to go into action again—giving the person unpredictable "trips"[3]—even years after the person has come off LSD.

---

3. **trips:** experiences or periods of euphoria, hallucination, etc., induced by a psychedelic drug, especially LSD.

This was an observable phenomenon—dramatically so!

In the face of this discovery, was it then also possible that residues of other drugs could lock up in the system and at some point reactivate with similar, if less dramatic, effect?

And if so, how did one then ever fully free people from the effects of drugs? Were they simply doomed thereafter to be at the effect of drugs whenever these residues chanced to reactivate?

What of the other debilitating effects of the presence of these drug residues? It was known that drugs burn up vitamin reserves. What other physical consequences might stem from the hidden presence of such drug deposits?

One could not ignore the possibility that, even when "dormant"[4]—if that expression can indeed ever be used for a toxic substance—they might be highly damaging to the organism.

And what of the potential spiritual and mental growth of individuals so affected? For it was also an observable fact that one was faced with some unchanging characteristics in a certain number of these cases, even when much of the mental and spiritual trauma of drug experiences had apparently been relieved. Among these characteristics was a "woodenness"[5] of personality and a noticeable difficulty in the ability to absorb and comprehend or retain and apply new data—in other words, an impaired ability to learn or change.

What was the answer to these cases?

---

4. **dormant:** in a state of rest or inactivity; inoperative.

5. **woodenness:** a condition of being without spirit, animation or awareness; being dull or stupid.

No known method existed for ridding the body of these minute drug deposits which, locked as they were in the tissues, were not totally dispelled in the normal processes of elimination.

The answer obviously did not lie in attempting to handle with more drugs or biochemicals which would only compound the situation.

But could a method be evolved to dislodge and flush them out, thereby freeing the person for full rehabilitation physically as well as mentally and spiritually?

The Original "Sweat Program"

Operating on the premise that the negative factors observed might be reversed if there were a means of getting LSD deposits out of the system, and that the most logical method to accomplish this would be to sweat them out, I worked out and released in 1977 a regimen called "The Sweat Program." Utilized mainly by those who had been heavily into drugs, particularly LSD, the procedure produced positive results. With it, evidences of the release of residues of other types of street drugs began to appear.

The regimen was a lengthy process, however, taking months to complete. A refinement and speed-up was needed.

Discovery of Other Embedded[6] Toxins

Using data and proven theories from earlier researches over the years, development was begun of a more comprehensive program, broader nutritionally and more streamlined.

---

6. **embedded:** having become fixed or incorporated, as into a surrounding mass.

From its earliest application another factor emerged which tended to support the theories upon which this new program was based: persons on the research program were reporting the apparent exudation[7] of substances other than just street drugs — substances smelling or tasting or feeling like medicines, anesthetics, diet pills, food preservatives, pesticides and any number of other chemical preparations in common use!

The list included not only LSD, heroin, cocaine, marijuana and "angel dust," but many other biochemical substances — medicinal and pharmaceutical drugs such as aspirin and codeine,[8] as well as commercial and agricultural and industrial chemicals.

These same persons were also experiencing, in mild form, some of the sensations of old sunburns, past illnesses and injuries and other past conditions, both physical and emotional.

Thus it seems that residues of any or all of these hostile biochemical substances apparently have the potential of remaining in the system, getting caught up in the tissues and remaining there, unsuspected, even after they have supposedly been eliminated from the body years earlier.

Their accumulation, unhandled, probably disarranges the biochemistry and fluid balance of the body.

This was my early thinking on the subject. It was now being borne out[9] by further research, as more and more

---

7. **exudation:** the action of coming out gradually in drops, as sweat, through pores or small openings; oozing out.

8. **codeine:** a narcotic derived from opium and resembling morphine, but less habit-forming: used for the relief of pain and in cough medicines.

9. **borne out:** substantiated; confirmed.

manifestations[10] occurred. (It has also since been borne out by clinical tests and by medical autopsies[11] which have found deposits of certain drugs embedded in body tissues.)

With the ongoing research, all indicators were that these substances were being flushed out as people progressed on the program. And these same individuals were reporting that they felt a new vigor, a renewed vitality and interest in life.

With a large number of people coming successfully through the regimen the research was completed.

The Purification program was released.

Elements of the Purification Program

The Purification program is a precisely designed regimen. It includes the following elements:

* Exercise, in the form of running, to stimulate the circulation.

* Prescribed periods in a sauna, which, accompanied by certain vitamins and other nutrients, enable one to sweat out the accumulated toxins.

* A nutritional program, including:

One's regular diet which is then supplemented with plenty of fresh vegetables which are not overcooked.

---

10. **manifestations:** outward or perceptible indications; materializations.

11. **autopsies:** inspections and dissections of bodies after death, as for determination of the cause of death; post-mortem examinations.

An exact regimen of vitamin, mineral and oil intake.

Sufficient liquids to offset the loss of body fluids through sweating.

A properly ordered personal schedule which provides the person with the normally required amount of sleep.

These are not unfamiliar actions to the majority of us.

How then can they accomplish what they apparently do? Why this particular set of actions? How is it that these elements, combined, might accomplish what no one of them apparently, singly or even in other combinations, has accomplished heretofore?[12]

While the procedures to be followed are not unusual, the answers to these questions lie in the very exact combination of the elements which make up the program, in the properties of the nutrients used in specific increments and in the increased proportions of these in exact ratio to each other, as laid out in detail in the next chapters of this book.

Warning

There is a warning which should be stressed in any description of this program. That is, simple and familiar as the outlined actions may appear:

They must be followed exactly for the best possible results.

---

12. **heretofore:** before this time; until now.

Because of the technical nature of the program, and because it is a strenuous program it must only be undertaken after a physical examination and written approval from an advised medical doctor.

Anyone with a weak heart or who is anemic[13] or who suffers from certain kidney conditions, for example, should not do this program but would require a similar but special program of a milder nature.

Additionally, while doing the program people have reported *re-experiencing* various effects of past drugs, medicine, alcohol or other stimulants or sedatives—including full-blown[14] drug "trips." For this reason, and for its success on any individual, it is best done under the close supervision of persons trained and experienced in its administration.

Also, even with this tight supervision, one does not do the actions by himself but always carries these out accompanied by a partner.

---

13. **anemic:** suffering from *anemia*, a condition in which there is a reduction of the number, or volume, of red blood cells or of the total amount of hemoglobin (the oxygen-carrying pigment of red blood cells that gives them their red color and serves to convey oxygen to the tissues) in the bloodstream, resulting in paleness, generalized weakness, etc.

14. **full-blown:** fully developed; complete.

3

How the Purification Program Works

3

How the Purification Program Works

How does the Purification program work?

Running is done to get the blood circulating deeper into the tissues where toxic residuals are lodged and thus act to loosen and release the accumulated harmful deposits and get them moving.

Very important, then, is that the running is immediately followed by sweating in the sauna to flush out the accumulations which have now been dislodged.

Regular nutrition and supplemental nutrition in the form of megavitamin[1] and mineral dosages and extra quantities of oil are a vital factor in helping the body to flush out toxins and to repair and rebuild the areas that have been affected by drugs and other toxic residuals.

A proper schedule with enough rest is mandatory, as the body will be undergoing change and repair throughout the program.

---

1. **megavitamin:** of, pertaining to or using very large amounts of vitamins.

These actions, carried out on a very stringently monitored basis, are apparently accomplishing a detoxification of the entire system, to the renewed health and vigor of the individual.

There is a more in-depth view to be taken of the entire process, however.

A person who has taken drugs, in addition to the physical factors involved, retains *mental image pictures* of those drugs and their effects. Mental image pictures are three-dimensional color pictures with sound and smell and all other perceptions, plus the conclusions or speculations of the individual. They are mental copies of one's perceptions sometime in the past. For example, a person who had taken LSD would retain "pictures" of that experience in his mind, complete with recordings of the sights, physical sensations, smells, sounds, etc., that occurred while he was under the influence of LSD.

Let us say an individual took LSD one day while at a fairground with some friends, and the day's experiences included feeling nauseated and dizzy, getting into an argument with a friend, feeling an emotion of sadness, and later feeling very tired. He would have mental image pictures of that entire incident.

Such mental image pictures can be reactivated by drug residuals, as the presence of these drugs in the tissues of the body can simulate the earlier drug experiences. This is known as *restimulation:* the reactivation of a past memory due to similar circumstances in the present approximating circumstances of the past.

Using the above example of the person who took LSD,

sometime later—perhaps years afterward—the residuals of the drug that are still in his body tissues can cause a restimulation of that LSD incident. The mental image pictures are reactivated, and he experiences the same sensations of nausea, dizziness and tiredness, and he feels sad. He does not know why. He might also perceive mental images of the persons he was with and the accompanying sights and sounds and smells.

Therefore, on the Purification program we are looking at two things: one, the actual drugs and toxic residuals in the body (and medical autopsies have shown that they are there); and two, the mental image pictures of the drugs and the mental image pictures of one's experiences with these drugs.

These two factors are hung up—one playing against the other, in perfect balance. What the person is feeling is the two conditions, one of them the actual presence of the drug residuals, the other the mental image pictures relating to them.

Probably the reason why the Purification program works is that it handles the one side of it—the accumulated toxic residuals—and thus fixes the person up so that the other side, the mental image picture side of it, is no longer in constant restimulation. It is as simple as that.

What, among other things, is happening on the Purification program is that you cause an upset of this perfect balance. Suddenly the balance isn't there anymore so you don't get the cross reaction anymore. The harmful and restimulative chemical residues have been flushed out—they're gone. This does not mean the mental image pictures are gone. But they are no longer in restimulation and they're not being reinforced by the presence of drug residuals.

Mental image pictures

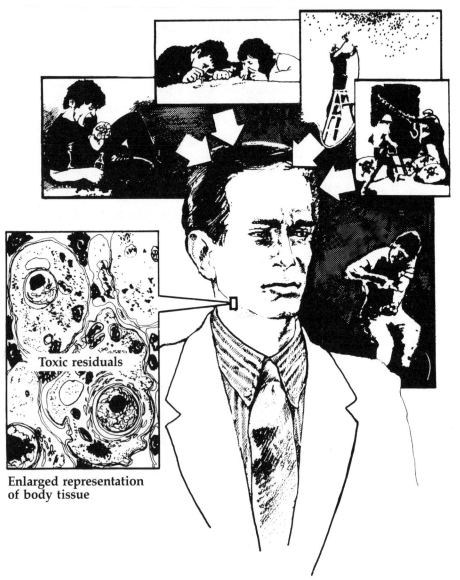

Toxic residuals

Enlarged representation
of body tissue

By breaking up the balance of these two and handling the one side of it on the Purification program we are restoring the person to better physical health and freeing him up as well for mental and spiritual gain.

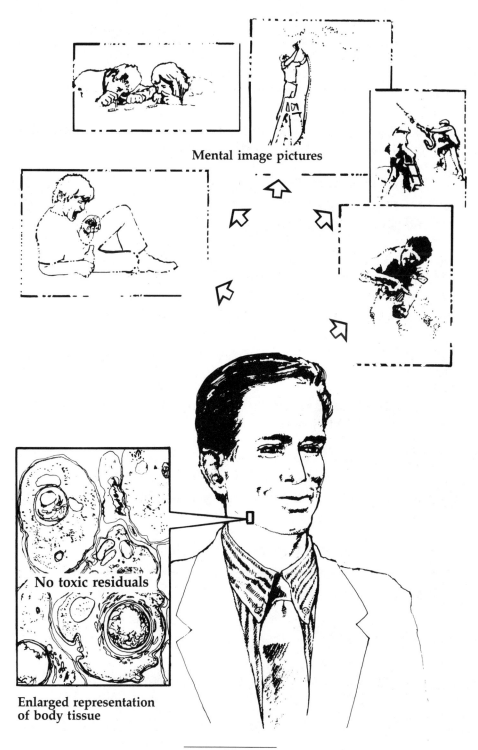

Mental image pictures

No toxic residuals

Enlarged representation
of body tissue

A "Long-Range Detoxification" Program

Drug residues can stop any mental help. They also stop a person's life! While originally addressed primarily to the handling of the accumulation of drugs in the system, it appears from the research results recorded and noted above that with use of this regimen many other toxic substances accumulated by the body can be flushed out of the system.

These substances must be eliminated if one is to get stable mental and spiritual improvement. The operating rule is that mental actions and even biophysical actions—methods of bringing an individual into better communication with his environment—do not work in the presence of life-hostile elements.

In rehabilitating an individual, only when we have accomplished a biochemical handling can we then go on to the next step, the biophysical handling (improving the person's ability to handle his body and environment) and then on to mental and spiritual improvement.

When one tries to move these around and put them out of sequence, one gets losses.

The development of a program to handle drugs and drug and chemical deposits in the body was based on the fact that successful rehabilitation of an individual can only be accomplished in the sequence outlined above.

Apparent gain occurs by cleaning up the body and can be seen as an end-all in itself, though that was not the original motivation.

In view of what it evidently accomplishes, the Purification program might be termed a long-range detoxification program. But it should be identified as itself, since it is unique among detoxification programs, both in its procedure and reported results. To my knowledge, there is no other known method by which these locked-in accumulations may be gotten out of the body.

4

Flushing Out Toxins

4

Flushing Out Toxins

On the Purification program, in order to flush the drugs and other toxins out of the body, a combination of *exercise*, in the form of running, and *sauna* is essential. These are done for a five-hour period daily, in a ratio of approximately:

twenty to thirty minutes of running, to
four to four and one-half hours sauna time.

The ratio is emphasized here as the bulk of the period is best spent in the sauna after the circulation has been worked up by running. In other words, the five-hour period is *not* 50 percent exercising and 50 percent sauna. The program gives best results with a much lower percentage of time exercising and a much higher percentage in the sauna.

Safeguard: Working with a Partner

Running and sauna sweatout should *always* be done with another person, as restimulation of past drugs, medicines, alcohol or even anesthetics can and does occur as the toxins get flushed out. This can include the restimulation of a full-blown "trip" from LSD or other drugs one may have taken.

Pairing up on the program so that one is *always* doing the running and sauna steps with a partner or even a third person, provides a safety factor in the case of any of the above eventualities.

Running

The first action on the program itself is running. The purpose of this is *not* to generate sweat but to get the blood circulating and the system functioning so that impurities held in the system can be released and pumped out.

Running increases the circulation throughout the whole body, thus:

a. it causes cell waste to be carried out more rapidly, and

b. it causes the circulation to go deeper into the muscles and tissues so that those areas which have been stagnant can now get rid of the accumulation of biochemical deposits and, in the case of LSD, the "residual crystals" which have been stored.

Running is done on a daily basis once the person has begun the program.

The running should be done on a gradient.[1] If one is so breathless that he can't talk to another while running then he is straining too much, so the running should be taken on a lower gradient.

---

1. **gradient:** a gradual approach to something taken step by step, level by level, each step or level being, of itself, easily surmountable—so that finally, quite complicated and difficult activities can be achieved with relative ease.

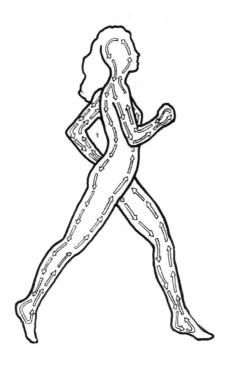

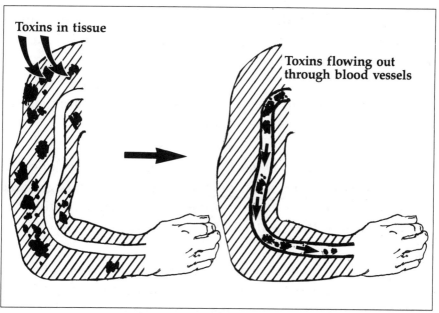

Toxins in tissue

Toxins flowing out
through blood vessels

Sweating in the Sauna

The second action, which directly follows the running, is sweating. A person goes into the sauna immediately after running in order to sweat. The impurities which have been freed up by the increased circulation can now be dispelled from the system and leave the body through the pores.

Sweating in the sauna is done at temperatures ranging anywhere from 140 degrees to 180 degrees. It is a matter of what temperature the person can take. Usually, but not always, a person beginning the program will start at a lower temperature and work up to a higher temperature. Then as he progresses he will find he can take increasing degrees of heat.

Clothing

Running is usually done in a regular sweat suit. This is optional, however, depending upon the geographical location, season or weather.

In the sauna one would simply wear a swimming suit or swimming trunks or some similar light apparel.

And, while it may seem almost absurd to include the following datum here, it has been included as the mistake was made (and swiftly corrected) in one area shortly following the initial release of the Purification program:

A sweat suit is *never* worn in the sauna. The reason for this is that a sweat suit acts as insulation, much the same as when a diver wears a wet suit for insulation against the cold of the sea.

Wearing a sweat suit would insulate one against the heat of the sauna and so inhibit and curtail[2] sweating.

Liquids

While on this program, it is important that one drink plenty of water, which greatly assists in flushing and cleansing the system. Additionally, with all the sweating done in the sauna it would be dangerous not to replenish body fluids. So a good amount of water, and any other nonalcoholic liquids the person might choose, should be taken daily.

Radiation and Liquids

On the Purification program, findings seem to bear out that there is a factor related to radiation that produces the greatest exudation of it and that is the sweating itself.

Radiation is apparently enormously water-soluble as well as water removable. According to researchers, one merely has to take a hose to a building surface or a road to wash the radiation off of it. This factor is well known to defense trained personnel.

So where one is doing the Purification program, one should be very careful to ensure that actual sweating occurs and in volume. A sufficient intake of water is therefore quite vital when doing the program.

This has a side effect, however, of washing a lot of minerals out of the system and perhaps vitamins, as well. Thus the intake of minerals and vitamins during the program is also a necessity.

---

2. **curtail:** cut short; reduce; abridge.

It is possible that the Purification program is not as workable when profuse sweating does not occur, when liquid intake is not large enough to compensate for it and when vitamins and minerals of a water-soluble nature are not carefully and adequately replaced. (The common vitamins taken on the Purification program which are not water-soluble are vitamins A,[3] D[4] and E.[5])

This gives us three important points which must be in on a Purification program:

1. Profuse sweating must occur.

2. A person's liquid intake must be large enough to compensate for the liquid lost through sweating.

3. Vitamins and minerals must be taken in sufficient quantities to replace those washed out of the system through sweating.

As megavitamin dosages are also a part of the Purification program, this mineral and vitamin intake is quite in addition to any other vitamin therapy ongoing at the time.

Overheating

One could get overheated in the sauna if it is not taken on the right gradient.

---

3. **A:** a vitamin important in bone growth, healthy skin, sexual function and reproduction.

4. **D:** a vitamin which is important in bone health and growth, calcium metabolism, nerve health and regulation of heartbeat.

5. **E:** a vitamin important in keeping oxygen from combining with waste products to form toxic compounds, and in red blood cell health.

When a person gets too warm or begins feeling faint, should the body temperature get too high, the recommendation is to go out and take a cool shower and then go back into the sauna. People who are having a hard time spending consecutive hours in the sauna will be able to handle the sauna time if a cooling shower is taken when needed.

Salt or Potassium[6] Depletion

Extra salt (sodium chloride) is not mandatory for every individual on the program. But salt and potassium are lost in sweating. Thus, one must watch for any symptoms of salt or potassium depletion and remedy the depletion at once, should it occur.

The symptoms can be similar to those of overheating or, when extreme, similar to the symptoms of heat exhaustion (clammy skin, extreme tiredness, weakness, headache and sometimes cramps, nausea, dizziness, vomiting or even fainting).

Such manifestations would be handled immediately with extra salt or salt tablets, potassium gluconate tablets, bioplasma,[7] or "salt substitute" which is mainly potassium.

A supply of these substances must be readily available at all times to anyone who is doing the Purification program. Ideally, supplies of these would be located right outside the sauna, clearly labeled as to what they are.

---

6. **potassium:** a mineral which helps to keep body fluids balanced and is important to the functioning of the nervous system.

7. **bioplasma:** a dietary supplement taken to replenish depleted supplies of various mineral salts naturally found in the body.

It is a matter of good common sense that overheating and salt or potassium depletion can be *prevented* by sufficient salt, potassium or bioplasma taken periodically while in the sauna and by cooling off when it becomes necessary during the sauna time. But should these symptoms occur, they must be handled and not considered something the person must "go through."

Also, one must guard against falling asleep in the sauna, as overheating or salt or potassium depletion could occur while one was asleep.

Salt or potassium depletion as a *chronic condition* must be handled as a separate factor by a medical doctor.

Heatstroke[8]

If perspiration ceases while in the sauna—the body suddenly stops sweating and the skin becomes hot and dry—it's an indicator[9] that needs immediate handling. This is a clamping down on the part of the body, a resistance to expelling, and it is the first sign of heatstroke.

The *Standard First Aid Personal Safety Booklet* put out by the American National Red Cross covers the symptoms of heat

---

8. **heatstroke:** a disturbance of the temperature-regulating mechanisms of the body caused by overexposure to excessive heat, resulting in fever, hot and dry skin and rapid pulse, sometimes progressing to delirium and coma.

9. **indicator:** a condition or circumstance arising during an action which indicates whether the action is running well or badly. A bad condition not getting any better or not lessening, or the person having losses would be *a bad indicator*. A bad condition getting better or becoming less present would be *a good indicator*. *Good indicators* also include such things as fast progress, person happy, having wins, etc.

exhaustion and/or heatstroke and the immediate aid to be given for such.

One would get the person out of the sauna at once and cool him off with a lukewarm or cool shower or sponging, or start with a lukewarm shower and gradually make it cooler. Fluids and salt, potassium or bioplasma would be given.

The first aid safety booklet must be kept on hand as a reference, readily available, in the sauna location.

Dry Sauna versus Wet Sauna

Thus far, the use of a dry sauna has proved to be the most successful in inducing profuse sweating in most people. It is possible that some may sweat more in a wet sauna; it has not yet been fully tested. It may be that it is an individual matter. There is no regulation on the program that outlaws the use of a wet sauna. Whichever type of sauna is employed, the whole idea is to use the system which permits the person to sweat the most.

Steam baths, at similar temperatures to the sauna, can be used by themselves when available. They serve much the same purpose as the dry sauna and it has been suggested that a steam bath may even work faster, but this has not been confirmed. The steam bath produces a similar effect. Thus, either can be used.

The same precautions apply to the use of a steam bath as to the sauna.

Eucalyptus[10] Oil

A small quantity of eucalyptus oil is sometimes added to the steam in a steam bath or similarly used in some saunas.

In a modern sauna or steam bath, the procedure is to simply put one or two capfuls of eucalyptus oil in a bucket of water in the room. As it then evaporates (the oil will evaporate before the water does), more can be added as needed.

Some people don't like the smell of eucalyptus at all, while others find it pleasant. If the solution is too strong it can cause watering of the eyes or nausea in some cases. Thus, one would survey before using it and, if used, it should be in appropriate small quantities.

Used correctly, eucalyptus has been reported to be beneficial in clearing up the lungs and clearing the sinuses. One person has reported his voice smoothing out as a result of using eucalyptus oil in the sauna.

It is not a mandatory step on the Purification program, but the data given here on the use of eucalyptus oil in the sauna or steam bath, as an optional element, should be known.

Whether or not eucalyptus is used, it goes without saying that a sauna or steam bath should be kept hygienic and free of odors by having the room scrubbed at least once, or oftener, daily.

---

10. **eucalyptus:** any of numerous often tall trees native to Australia and adjacent islands, having aromatic evergreen leaves that are the source of medicinal oils and heavy wood used as timber.

5

Importance of a Proper Schedule

5

Importance of a Proper Schedule

The properly ordered personal schedule required while one is on the Purification program consists of:

a. a sufficient amount of sleep daily.

b. correct ratio of running time to sauna time, and the total prescribed period for these adhered to daily.

c. sticking to the program sensibly and not skipping days or skimping or short-cutting on the pre-scribed daily schedule, nor doing any part of the program in a random fashion.

Ideally, this includes getting in the exercise (run-ning) and sauna time at approximately the same time each day; and taking the vitamin and mineral nutrients at approximately the same time each day, as when these factors are kept in predictably the program goes much more smoothly.

Sleep

The need for adequate sleep should be emphasized here as it has been found to be a vital, vital factor in the application of the program. People function best when they are sufficiently rested.

Eight hours of sleep is considered the usual daily requirement. Some persons may need more than this, but getting less than the regular amount of sleep one usually requires is not advised.

Some tiredness has not been uncommon at certain intervals during the course of the program even when the procedure was being carried out totally standardly. It can occur when the individual first goes onto the program and is not up to doing a five-hour stint[1] per day, in which case the person should build up to the full daily period on a gradient by doing a bit more time each successive day until he is able to do the full five hours. It can also occur as part of the restimulation in connection with medical or street drug residues or as part of the restimulation of an old illness, etc., any of which the person might run through while on this program. There are cases on record of persons going through periods of tiredness or fatigue connected with past illness and/or medical or drug experiences and coming through them far brighter and more energetic.

But it must be borne in mind that the Purification program can be strenuous. Trying to do it on too little sleep would be a severe violation of the regulations covering the program. A person obviously needs enough sleep and rest in order to cope with the changes taking place in his body and in order to assist the body in any needed rebuild of tissues or cellular repair. Per

---

1. **stint:** a period of time spent doing something.

Program Case Supervisor[2] reports, where a schedule for sufficient sleep has been violated the person has often wound up having a rough time of it, which is totally unnecessary. Quite apart from any mere tiredness, any reactions which are there to be restimulated by drug residues can, due to insufficient sleep and rest, produce unnecessary and nonoptimum reactions.

One obviously cannot expect to make the gains that are possible on the Purification program unless this point is in.

Optimum Daily Time on the Program

From the many cases interviewed and from data from those who have supervised the program, five hours exercise and sauna daily has been found to be ideal for the majority of people doing the Purification program. The program apparently works like a bomb[3] when the highest percentage of this time is spent in the sauna and a lesser percentage in running. (Example: A good ratio has been found to be approximately 20 to 30 minutes of running to get the circulation up, followed by the remainder of the time spent in the sauna, for a total of five hours.)

Not everyone has gone immediately onto a full five-hour stint right from the start. (And some have successfully done the program on a shorter daily schedule.)

In both the running and the sauna, where the right gradient was applied—particularly when beginning the program—it went very smoothly.

---

2. **Program Case Supervisor:** that person assigned the responsibility of overseeing the delivery of and ensuring the proper and exact application of all aspects of the Purification program to individual *cases*—persons being treated or helped.

3. **works like a bomb:** does something extremely well.

Age and Physical Condition–Factors in Scheduling

Age, physical condition and stamina can all enter into it, and these factors would need to be taken into consideration for each program participant individually when starting the person on the program.

Among the many people surveyed on program results were those who had required a few days to work up to five hours daily. However, once up to the five-hour daily schedule, that proved to be the optimum daily period for those persons, as it has for so many of the people who have been through the program.

Additionally, on such a schedule the Purification program can and has been completed effectively in the shortest possible amount of time.

Most people approached the five-hour daily program eagerly and enthusiastically.

Some eager beavers were found apt to plunge in a bit too quickly at the start, and this was handled by having them work up gradually to where they could run 20 to 30 minutes without strain while at the same time increasing the sauna time gradually up to the full prescribed period.

One Program Case Supervisor reported a few people staying in the sauna too long with no break and turning on[4] headaches and other unnecessary reactions as a result. The purpose should not be to see how long one can stay in the sauna for any one stretch of time—and this had to be clarified with several such enthusiasts.

---

4. **turning on:** starting suddenly to affect or show.

What worked best was when the person had been in the sauna sweating for a while and had a good sweat going and then came out, got some fresh air and space and cooled off, as needed. Then he or she went right back into the sauna for more sweating. When plenty of liquids (many people take water jugs into the sauna with them) and enough salt, potassium and bioplasma were used, the sauna time went very well.

How Long Does the Purification Program Take?

With each of the points of the program kept in and the regimen followed exactly, the program can be completed by many at five hours a day in two or three weeks time.

Some persons may take a bit more time than that; a few might complete the program in less time.

6

Nutrition

6

Nutrition

Nutrition plays a vital role in the Purification program. But when we speak of nutrition in relation to the program we are not talking only about food in the most common usage of the word. We are talking about vitamins and minerals as well.

Regular Eating Habits

There are *no* "special diets" required on this program.

The person simply eats what he normally would, supplemented with plenty of vegetables which have not been overcooked and with the recommended dosages of vitamins and minerals.

There is no thought here of putting the person on any kind of special diet at all. There are no restrictions on what one may eat. We are not even trying to preach against toxic foods or campaign against diet abuses or junk foods or anything of that sort.

We are only trying to handle the *accumulation* of impurities built up in the body. If one wanted to defend his body against all future impurities then that is another program and not part of this one.

To put a person on a diet different than that to which he is accustomed is to introduce a sudden change in the midst of other changes he will be experiencing on the program. A change of diet might be just one too many changes and would be an additive[1] which could interfere with and affect the efficacy of the program.

Diets and Food Fads

I am not a food faddist and there is no idea of mixing any food fad into this program. However, there is plenty of food faddism going on in society and you can easily start such a fad, so this must be watched when administering the Purification program. There is no intention to have people eating banana fronds split into diamonds and star shapes and blessed by some deity[2] or other, or a fad of "three lettuce leaves criss-crossed with two slabs of peanut butter as an absolute must eighteen times a day," or something equally silly being touted[3] as "the only food a person can have."

Food is subject to becoming very faddist and, frankly, most people know very little about it.

---

1. **additive:** a thing which has been added. This usually has a bad meaning in that an *additive* is said to be something needless or harmful which has been done in addition to standard procedure. *Additive* normally means a departure from standard procedure. For example, someone administering the Purification program puts different or additional nutritional requirements into the basic lineup called for by the program. It means a twist on standard procedure. In common English, *additive* might mean a substance put into a compound to improve its qualities or suppress undesirable qualities. In this book it definitely means to add something to the technical procedure resulting in undesirable results.

2. **deity:** a god or goddess.

3. **touted:** described or advertised boastfully; publicized or promoted; praised extravagantly.

Locating and remedying deficiencies and excesses in vitamins, minerals, enzymes,[4] sugar, protein, oil and fats, carbohydrates and bulk fiber[5] as well as other dietary supplements is the keynote of dieting. No special substance or food or abstinence from it is a whole answer.

Diets should be considered a subject where one seeks a balance of body support elements and determines quantity.

Fasting,[6] magic foods eaten to the exclusion of others and dozens of dietary fads alike tend to be more harmful than beneficial.

There is a vast difference between food-faddism and the subject of diets. Diets have become viewed as what a person is *limited to* in eating, whereas they should be viewed as what a person *must have* as nutritional elements. This has become a problem because the true natural diet of man has not been isolated.

Theory of a Natural Diet

Food, lack of it, incorrect planning or consumption of it or substitution or alteration of it can vastly affect health.

Man is not a primary converter of natural energy or masses but depends upon other converters for a primary conversion in most cases. (Except for vitamin D and one or two

---

4. **enzymes:** complex organic substances secreted by certain cells of plants and animals which cause a chemical change in the substance upon which they act.

5. **fiber:** the structural part of plants and plant products that consists of carbohydrates that are wholly or partially indigestible and when eaten helps to move waste products through the intestines.

6. **fasting:** abstaining from all food.

other items man, for instance, does not convert sunlight to energy, but, eating algae[7] which does so convert, is able to obtain and use the energy.)

No real study of or search for the natural diet of man has ever been made or attempted. Studies are made of diets from the viewpoint of how to correct illnesses or maintain health but not what the basic food of the human body would be. Scarcities, availabilities, what can be grown and preserved, the ease of growing, climatic and soil and water conditions, and how to make a profit are factors which have established diet instead of "What does the human body require?"

The human body is a complex biological carbon-oxygen engine, one running at an operating temperature of 37 degrees centigrade[8] and, being biological, has the ability to establish and repair itself. To its food requirements then are added the elements required to build as well as to run the body.

Almost all mammals live about six times their period of growth. Man lives only three and one-third times his growth period. As other mammals than man are under the same or greater stress, but are usually uniform in diet while healthy, it can be assumed that man has departed from his natural diet.

Some guesses have been made as to natural diet by an examination of teeth but this would not be an adequate approach.

---

7. **algae:** a group of plants, either one-celled or many-celled, often growing in colonies. Algae contain chlorophyll (the green coloring matter of plants) and other pigments, but have no true root, stem or leaf. They are found in water or damp places and include seaweed, pond scum, etc.

8. **centigrade:** pertaining to or noting a temperature scale in which 0 degrees represents the ice point and 100 degrees the steam point. Also called *Celsius*.

The resolution of man's natural diet as opposed to what he is eating might do a very great deal to improving racial health.

Man's mass efforts towards diet are targeted for quantity and profit. Efforts to establish quality are often resisted by various special interests in the mistaken idea that further knowledge of diet might reduce quantity and profit. However, it could be that new food discoveries would vastly increase both production quantity potential and profit.

No simple basis for research and discovery of the natural diet exists in known statement form. The necessary first steps to the discovery of man's correct diet would be:

a. The statement of a possibility that one might have existed or did exist.

b. A formula for search and possible discovery of it.

This section of the book has made (a) above.

The following would be a formula for its discovery:

Overweight: Residual elements of food, substances or gases which are not totally eliminated or utilized by the body after ingestion.

Underweight or debility:[9] Inadequate or lacking foods, substances or gases which are needed for the activity, maintenance or repair of the body.

By listing all foods, substances or gases which are *stored* by

---

9. **debility:** weakness or feebleness, especially of the body.

the body, one would obtain a list of things ingested, part of which were not utilized or necessary. Simple recording of those items which put on unwanted weight would be a part of this action. The examination of overweight persons and their diets would give another section of it. Further examination of cadavers[10] that had been overweight would round out the list. Which of these were the result of body conversion of what food would be noted.

A study and listing of all deficiency diseases and malnutrition cases as contained in *The Textbook of Medicine,* Beeson and McDermott, and in other papers and texts would give a list of items vital to the activity, maintenance and repair of the body.

The items in the overweight and debility lists could then be compared.

One would have, as a result, the elements of a natural diet.

A search for foods which contained *only* the elements which were *used* and *vital* could be undertaken.

The result would be the elements of a possible natural diet.

An examination of the ease of production and supply of such foods could then result in a practical natural diet.

Zonal application in specific areas might require the repetition of the formula to take in racial or climatic or production variables.

---

10. **cadavers:** dead bodies, especially human bodies to be dissected; corpses.

It is said that 80 percent of Americans are overweight. Their activity and intelligence are failing. The populations of many countries are starving or suffering malnutrition.

The wild animals, fish and fowl are ceasing to be a world source of food supply. There is no reason to go on killing off all life on the planet simply because no one knows, beyond opinion or taste, what man's natural food was or could be.

Fads and hobbies should not be the sole source of data on this subject.

The problem could be intelligently solved and should be if we are still to have a populated planet.

Probably the planet could support billions more than it does. Most of it is wasteland.

A system to solve it by killing off populations through sterilizing and euthanasia[11] is simply impractical, stupid and useless suppression.

It would be far better to work out man's natural diet.

This is quite another subject of research which could be undertaken by others whose primary field it is, but the discovery of such basics and making these widely known could result in a planet-wide program which would at some future time

---

11. **euthanasia:** the original definition of *euthanasia* is "mercy killing," the act of putting to death painlessly or allowing to die (as by withholding extreme medical measures) a person or animal suffering from an incurable disease or condition. However, under the practice of psychiatry it has become "the act of killing people considered a burden on society."

decidedly augment the basic principles and implementation of the Purification program.

Meantime, it is not intended that dietary fads of any sort be included as part of the Purification program.

7

Oil: Trading Bad Fat for Good Fat

7

Oil: Trading Bad Fat for Good Fat

Toxic substances seem to lock up mainly, but not exclusively, in the fat tissues of the body.

The theory is that one could replace the fat tissues that hold these accumulations with fat tissue which is free of such residues. It is a theory of exchange. It is based on the "Have–Waste" theory and formulas from my research in the 1950s, as described below.

Have–Waste Theory

Havingness is a term for a very fundamental principle which can be seen in operation in several different aspects of the Purification program.

Havingness has to do with a person's considerations[1] in regard to mass. It means, to state it simply, the degree to which

---

1. **considerations:** thoughts or beliefs about something.

one is willing to experience mass—mass of any kind. One's degree of havingness is the degree that he is able to *have* or *not have* a particular thing, with no compulsion involved either way.

In good shape, a being should be able to experience anything. His recorded experience, however, may dictate otherwise.

His level of havingness is actually determined by his considerations on the subject. And his considerations can be influenced by a combination of factors, past and present. But the basic influencing factors in this are abundance and scarcity.

There is a little scale in operation here which was put to extensive test early in my work with people. While its application is broad, the simplicity of the scale, or formula, is just this:

> Before a being can *have* something, he must be able to *waste* it.

If an individual can't *have* something, it is a cinch[2] he'll *waste* it. And if he can't even waste it, it is a cinch he'll *substitute* for it.

We use this principle on the Purification program to effect the exchanges which are needed.

While the research and formulas of "Have–Waste" go very

---

2. **cinch:** (*slang*) something that is sure to happen or easy to do.

extensively into the subjects of being able to have, being able to waste and other aspects of these conditions, a very simple premise on which this theory can be explained is that:

Anything which is scarce becomes valuable.

The body will actually tend to hold onto something it is short of. Thus, if you try to get rid of something it is short of, it will resist giving it up.

The answer is to provide an additional supply of the substance.

Therefore, in the matter of fat, if the person takes some oil the body might possibly exchange the bad fat in the body for the good oil. That is the basic theory.

I am also indebted for material on this to a doctor in Portugal who, in conversation, told me that autopsies had found all sorts of grisly, used-up fat stored in unlikely places in people's bodies. In other words, there is a lot of unusable fat a body can accumulate.

The body will obviously hold onto a lot of fat and won't let go of it. The effort is to get the body to take good oil or fat in exchange for the bad, toxin-ridden fat it is holding onto. If one wants somebody to clean up the fat tissue in the body, he had better give the body some fat in order to make up for the fat tissues the body is now, on the Purification program, releasing or changing.

In this way we have some chance of getting the body to release fatty tissue which is impregnated[3] with toxic substances. We get the body to trade fat for fat.

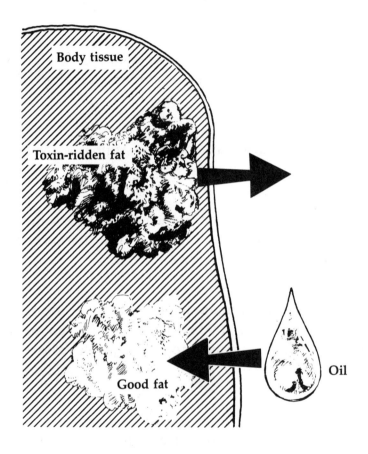

Oils

One should use a blend of oils which contains soy, walnut, peanut and safflower oil.

---

3. **impregnated:** infused or permeated throughout, as with a substance; saturated.

Whether purchasing the oil in a health food or other type of store one should ensure it is fresh, not rancid.

If this type of oil is not obtainable in health food stores or elsewhere, one could blend it from these four oils in the proper amounts. Any oil used must be cold-pressed[4] and polyunsaturated,[5] and must be kept refrigerated so it remains fresh.

The oil used on the program must also include lecithin.[6] Lecithin appears to be an agent capable of breaking fat into tiny particles which can pass readily into the tissues. It should be taken along with the oil on the Purification program, and is obtainable from most health food stores in a granulated form. The amount of lecithin to be taken has been estimated to be between one and two tablespoons per day, depending on how much oil one is taking. In its granulated form, it can be mixed with other food such as milk, yogurt or juice.

How Much Oil?

Upon initial release of the Purification program, the exact daily quantity of oil needed by a person on the program had not been definitely established, beyond the fact that it was very likely somewhere between two tablespoonfuls and one-half

---

4. **cold-pressed:** produced through extraction by pressure without the use of heat.

5. **polyunsaturated:** a kind of fat or oil that (unlike animal or dairy fats) is not associated with the formation of cholesterol (a fatty substance associated with hardening of the arteries) in the blood.

6. **lecithin:** a complex fatty substance which is found in egg yolk and contains phosphorus (a mineral which helps give strength to bones and aids in metabolism).

cup, depending upon the individual. One tablespoon of oil is not going to accomplish much, as too little oil won't let the body substitute good fat tissue for bad. If too much is given it can cause diarrhea.

A medical doctor who has handled numerous people on the program has reported that the most standard oil dosage found to be required by most persons he supervised on the program was between two and four tablespoonfuls a day. Others, particularly some 250-pounders under his care on the program, were on considerably more oil than that.

The recommendation of this medical doctor is that on an oil dosage of any quantity, one would reduce the oil intake if the oil showed up in a bowel movement or in the body sweat, as in such case there is an excess of oil which is not being put to use but simply expelled.

One way to test whether the person is on the right amount of oil would be to put him on a scale daily and keep a close check on his weight. (This should be done routinely, in any event, when a person is on the Purification program.) If the fat is being replaced in the body, then the weight will not go up despite the intake of oil. If the body is simply assimilating the oil, with no exchange in fat tissue, the weight will increase. Such a change in weight would tend to indicate the body was simply adding new fat tissue rather than exchanging old fat tissue for new fat tissue.

Evening Primrose Oil

Evening primrose oil is the oily extract from the crushed seeds of the evening primrose plant. According to researchers, it purportedly handles various food allergies and furnishes a substance which seems to help break down dietary fat and fatty tissue. It is available in many health food stores in capsule form.

Pilots[7] done on the use of evening primrose oil on the Purification program have shown that it appears to benefit persons with a history of an inability to metabolize fat (as evidenced by a lack of weight loss when moderately dieting), and persons with heavy drug or alcohol histories. Persons on these pilots were given six capsules (500 mg. each) of evening primrose oil per day—three capsules twice a day with meals—in addition to the usual amounts of oil on the program.

Occasionally persons with a history of an inability to metabolize fat would seem to do better if the amount of evening primrose oil was increased to nine or twelve capsules per day and the regular oil dosage was reduced one tablespoon from what would be a normal dose for that person.

One medical doctor reported that evening primrose oil also seemed to assist persons who had trouble metabolizing the normal dosages of oil on the Purification program. Although this is not a common occurrence, this doctor found that when such a person was given six capsules of evening primrose oil per day along with the normal oil dosage on the program, the person was usually able to handle the oil.

All Bodies Have Some Fatty Tissue

All people, be they fat or thin, have some fatty tissue in the body. Some, of course, have more fat stored in their bodies than others. On this program we simply want to get rid of the fat that

---

7. **pilots:** preliminary or experimental trials or tests.

contains the toxic substances. We are not trying to make people lose weight.

Worth mentioning here, also, and of interest to thin people, is the fact that while toxic substances lock up mainly in fat tissue it does not mean that the person cannot have drug deposits in other tissues.

Taking the Oil

Some individuals reported difficulty taking the oil by itself, usually due more to the texture than to the actual taste.

As there seemed to be no reason why the oil could not be taken in orange juice or mixed with some other food of the person's choice and taken that way, this was the handling used for those persons who had difficulty getting the oil down. This gave good results, *provided* the entire dosage of oil was consumed. Others simply took the oil alone. (In taking the oil dosage mixed with other food, the exception is that one would *not* cook food in the oil and then consider that *that* was the oil ration for the day!)

When to Take the Oil

On the initial program, the oil dosage was taken at the same time as one of the regular meals.

One doctor has suggested that, as the oil may coat the stomach and intestinal walls for a certain period (which could prevent the assimilation of other nutrients, especially the water-soluble vitamins), the oil is probably best taken before going to bed or at least at a different mealtime than when the vitamins and minerals are taken. This was not put to stringent test on the program and many participants did well when taking both oil and vitamins at the same meal. The suggestion is included here as a point for consideration in a case where it appears the individual is not getting the full benefit that would be expected from the recommended vitamin dosages.

Adequate Oil Is Essential

Adequate oil intake is essential to successful implementation of the program. One could not expect the desired results from the Purification program without a sufficient amount of oil on a daily basis.

And the oil *must* be pure and stored properly so that it does not become rancid.

Oils Can Go Rancid

Apparently oils such as those used on the Purification program can go rancid after a period of time and can also go rancid if they are improperly stored or subjected to heat.

This includes combinations of soy, safflower, peanut and walnut oils, vitamin A, vitamin D, vitamin E and wheat germ oil.

According to published nutritional research, rancid fats (oils) destroy important vitamins in the body and this can eventually result in a physical condition of swollen joints or cords[8] or muscles, known as "gout."[9]

---

8. **cords:** tendons: any of the inelastic cords of tough, fibrous connective tissue in which muscle fibers end and by which muscles are attached to bones or other parts; sinews.

9. **gout:** an acute, recurrent disease characterized by painful inflammation of the joints, chiefly those in the feet and hands, and especially in the big toe, and by an excess of uric acid (a white, odorless substance found in urine) in the blood.

Wheat Germ Oil

An example is wheat germ oil. If you look at a bottle of vitamin E you will see that it is mainly wheat germ oil. Apparently wheat germ oil, after being pressed, will only last a week before it goes rancid. Taking this oil after it has gone rancid could bring about, after exercise, agonizing cramps (or in severe cases, the condition of gout).*

If a person took rancid wheat germ oil while on the Purification program he might incorrectly attribute these sore muscles to the exercise, when in actual fact it was the result of the rancidity of the oil.

Rancidity in Other Oils

One could find oil in other places that has turned rancid—such as that contained in mayonnaise that has not been properly refrigerated.

According to Adelle Davis,[10] some manufacturers even use rancid oils in the preparation of margarines, cooking fats and highly refined commercial vegetable oils. She recommends that one consume only cold-pressed, unrefined oils. And even these must be stored properly or they can turn rancid.

Storage of Oils

Apparently one factor that can cause these oils to go rancid is exposure to the sun or radiation. One person in charge of the

* There are recommended dietary handlings for a person who has gout in the book *Let's Get Well*, by Adelle Davis, published by Harcourt Brace Jovanovich, Inc. Any person who does have what appears to be a condition of gout should consult a qualified medical practitioner. —Editor

10. **Adelle Davis:** prominent American nutritionist, author of books on nutrition, including *Let's Eat Right to Keep Fit, Let's Cook It Right, Let's Have Healthy Children* and *Let's Get Well.*

Purification program in an area reported that a jar of vitamin E, left out in the sun, went rancid within a matter of days. And if a bottle of oil, or a container of oil capsules (such as those in which vitamin A, D and E are often sold), is stored for a long period of time instead of being used up, it could go rancid.

The best thing to do is to keep these oils in a refrigerator and test them periodically to ensure none of them have turned rancid.

How to Detect Rancid Oil

The simplest way to tell if an oil has gone rancid is to smell it. Rancid oil smells peculiar—it does not smell at all like the same oil when fresh.

With a bottle of oil such as that used on the Purification program (a blend of four oils), one just needs to open the bottle and smell it. And with capsules of oil, such as vitamin E capsules, you can simply poke a hole in one of the capsules and smell the oil to see if it is rancid.

Other Forms

Vitamins A, D and E can be obtained in dry tablet form and it is quite okay for persons on the Purification program to take these in place of oil capsules of the specific vitamin. The advised dosage would not change.

One does, however, need to take the recommended *oil* dosage in its oil form, and this should be a blend of the four oils—soy, walnut, peanut and safflower—plus lecithin. The intake of oil is an essential part of the Purification program in order to effect the exchange of fat for fat.

With vitamins, the important point is protecting them from sunlight, heat and oxygen—therefore vitamin containers should be kept closed and stored in a refrigerator. There is no reason one could not take vitamins such as A, D and E in oil capsule form as long as they are properly stored and not permitted to go rancid.

In summary, certain oils are essential to the effectiveness of the Purification program, and thus it is vital that adequate measures are taken to ensure that none of these oils are rancid.

This is done by:

1. Proper storage of oils, including not only bottled oils but also those oils contained in capsules, such as vitamin E. Oils should be kept refrigerated and not left out in the sunlight or near any heat.

2. Oils should be checked regularly to see if they have turned rancid.

3. Any oils that are rancid should be thrown out as soon as rancidity is detected.

Research findings point to the possibility that rancid oils are a health hazard of a magnitude not previously suspected. Oils used in cooking or commercial processing of food, where they are not fresh, pure and free of rancidity, have been linked with digestive and muscular ills and even cancer.

One sees, therefore, the importance of ensuring that only fresh, nonrancid oil is used, in one's daily living as well as on the Purification program.

8

Calcium and Magnesium: The "Cal-Mag Formula"

8

Calcium and Magnesium: The "Cal-Mag Formula"

Although both calcium and magnesium are included in the multimineral tablet used on the program, additional dosages of these are an integral part of the program because of their particular effectiveness in helping to handle the effects of drugs.

Calcium: A Basic Building Block

Calcium is a must where any healing or exchange process is involved, as it is a basic building block.

More important, it is calcium that affects the nervous system.[1]

I do not know the total relationship between calcium and toxic substances (and neither, apparently, does anyone else) but it actually exists.

The rationale back of this is that calcium in deficiency sets a person up for spasms. Nerve spasms occur in the absence of calcium; muscular spasms are caused by lack of calcium. A person who thinks he is in a state of high tension or something of the sort may simply have a calcium deficiency.

---

1. **nervous system:** the system of nerves and nerve centers in an animal or human, including the brain, spinal cord, nerves and masses of nerve tissue.

Calcium and Magnesium in Tandem[2]

Calcium would be administered in company with magnesium. Nervous reactions are diminished with magnesium; magnesium itself has proven necessary to keep the nerves smoothed out. Both calcium and magnesium are helpful in preventing sore muscles. But they are best administered together in a specific ratio.

Calcium Needs an Acidic Base

In pairing up these two minerals, the main factor to be resolved in order to obtain positive benefit from calcium dosages was this: Calcium does not go into solution in the body and is not utilized unless it is in an acid. That is the odd thing about calcium—it has to have an acidic base in which to operate.

And magnesium is alkaline.[3]

If the system is too alkaline the calcium will not release the positive ion[4] which makes it possible for the calcium to operate in the cellular structure and go through the blood vessel walls and the intestinal walls and so forth. In other words, in an alkaline system, calcium is ineffective and inactive. Thus, some sort of resolution was required.

Development of the "Cal-Mag Formula"

Working on the use of calcium and magnesium in 1973 for purposes other than the handling of drug reactions, I found a means of getting calcium into solution in the body along with magnesium so that the benefits of both could be achieved. The

2. **tandem:** a relationship between two persons or things involving cooperative action, mutual dependence, etc.

3. **alkaline:** of or like the class of substances that neutralize and are neutralized by acids, and form caustic or corrosive solutions in water.

4. **ion:** an electrically charged atom or group of atoms formed by the loss or gain of one or more electrons. A positive ion is created by electron loss, and a negative ion is created by electron gain.

answer was to add vinegar, which would provide the acidic formula needed.

The result was a solution which proved to be highly effective, which was named the "Cal-Mag Formula."

Calcium-Magnesium Ratio

The proven ratio used in the Cal-Mag Formula is one part elemental magnesium to two parts elemental calcium.

As the Cal-Mag Formula calls for precise amounts of these elemental substances, some further explanation of these quantities should be given here.

The Cal-Mag Formula is made using the compounds calcium gluconate and magnesium carbonate. Both of these come in white, powdery form. Each is a compound of different substances. In other words, calcium gluconate contains other substances besides calcium; it is not all pure calcium but contains only a percentage of pure elemental calcium. Similarly, magnesium carbonate contains other substances besides magnesium, and includes only a percentage of pure elemental magnesium.

But it is the amount of elemental magnesium in correct ratio to the amount of elemental calcium that is important in the preparation of the Cal-Mag Formula. This does *not, not, not* mean that you use pure magnesium or pure calcium when you make Cal-Mag. Use only calcium gluconate and magnesium carbonate.

Magnesium Carbonate: The desired compound for Cal-Mag, called magnesium carbonate basic, contains 29 percent magnesium. (This compound is also sometimes called magnesium alba.)

There are different magnesium compounds with different percentages of elemental magnesium, but using any kind other than that recommended here will give varying amounts of magnesium which will violate the needed ratio of one part magnesium to two parts calcium.

It is magnesium carbonate basic, containing 29 percent elemental magnesium which is used in making Cal-Mag. And it is essential to ensure that the magnesium carbonate basic which is used is fresh, not old.

Calcium Gluconate: There is only one kind of calcium gluconate compound and 9 percent of that compound is calcium, so there is no problem in selecting the correct calcium gluconate compound for the Cal-Mag preparation.

The Cal-Mag Formula

The Cal-Mag Formula, as released in the early 1970s, is repeated here.

Note, again, that the ratio is one part elemental magnesium to two parts elemental calcium. If one wants to work this out precisely, one can work out the elemental amounts. The formula below has been given for the compound amounts.

1. Put 1 level tablespoon of calcium gluconate in a normal-sized drinking glass.

2. Add ½ level teaspoon of magnesium carbonate.

3. Add 1 tablespoon of cider vinegar (at least 5 percent acidity).

4. Stir it well.

5. Add ½ glass of boiling water and stir until all the powder is dissolved and the liquid is clear. (If this doesn't occur it could be from poor grade or old magnesium carbonate.)

6. Fill the remainder of the glass with lukewarm or cold water and cover.

The solution will stay good for two days.

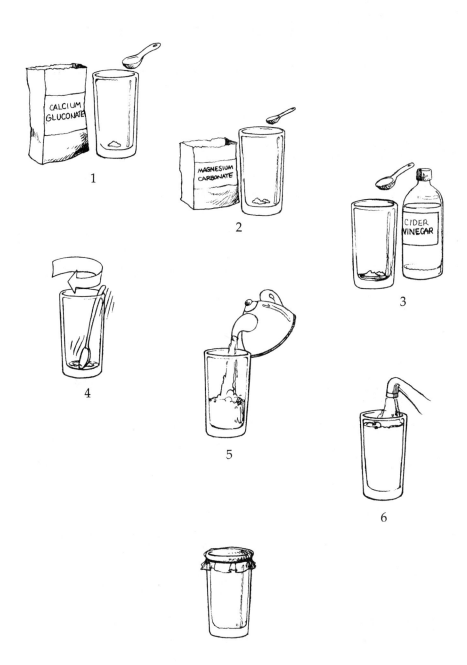

1

2

3

4

5

6

Metric System Equivalents

Another statement of the quantity of each component of Cal-Mag could be made.

By the terms *tablespoon* and *teaspoon* is meant the standard household capacity measures used in the English system of weights and measures. These are precise measures and should not be confused with the eating utensils of the same names. (Besides being imprecise as measuring spoons, the names of such eating utensils mean different capacities in different parts of the world. For example, a "tablespoon" *eating utensil* in Australia is twice the size of a "tablespoon" *eating utensil* in the United States.)

For parts of the world which do not use the English system of weights and measures, the metric system equivalents will clear up any possible question as to the proportions to be used in the formula.

One tablespoon per the English system of weights and measures = 15 milliliters (14.8 ml. to be exact) per the metric system.

One teaspoon per the English system of weights and measures = 5 milliliters (4.9 ml. to be exact) per the metric system.

These figures can be rounded off because the differences are so slight as to be negligible, and by rounding them off they remain in correct ratio.

Substituting these metric equivalents would give a Cal-Mag Formula as follows:

1. Put 15 ml. calcium gluconate in a normal-sized drinking glass.

2. Add 2.5 ml. magnesium carbonate.

3. Add 15 ml. of cider vinegar (at least 5 percent acidity).

4. Stir it well.

5. Add ½ glass (or about 120 ml.) of boiling water and stir until all the powder is dissolved and the liquid is clear. (If this doesn't occur it could be from poor grade or old magnesium carbonate.)

6. Fill the remainder of the glass with lukewarm or cold water and cover.

Graduated cylinders with milliliter increments marked on them are available from laboratory supply houses in different sizes, so one can get accurate measures whether a single glass or a large batch of Cal-Mag is to be made.

Important: Make a Palatable[5] Cal-Mag

There is a warning regarding Cal-Mag. Variations from the above can produce an unsuccessful mess that can taste pretty horrible. It can be made incorrectly so that it doesn't dissolve

---

5. **palatable:** acceptable or agreeable to the sense of taste.

and become the most unpalatable, ghastly stuff anybody ever fed anybody. Possibly when made incorrectly it is even unworkable.

There is also the factor that one should mix the solution in exactly the correct proportions and approach the dosage on the cautious side, as an overdose of magnesium can cause diarrhea. I doubt, however, that as much as three glasses of properly mixed Cal-Mag would bring about that condition.

Made correctly, Cal-Mag is a very clear liquid, pleasant to take and palatable. Thus the directions should be followed very explicitly, to produce a proper Cal-Mag that is both pleasant to take and beneficial.

Cal-Mag has been found to have the added benefit of balancing out the vitamin B_1[6] used on the program, as vitamin B_1 taken without calcium can cause serious teeth problems by setting up an imbalance of vitamins and minerals.

---

6. **vitamin B_1:** a vitamin, also called thiamine, important to the body in the functions of cell oxidation (respiration), growth, carbohydrate metabolism, stimulation and transmission of nerve impulses, etc.

9

Niacin,
the "Educated"
Vitamin

9

Niacin, the "Educated" Vitamin

Niacin,[1] as one of the B complex[2] vitamins, is essential to nutrition. It is so vital to the effectiveness of the Purification program that it requires some extensive mention here.

It can produce some startling, and in the end very beneficial, results when taken properly on the program along with the other necessary vitamins and minerals in sufficient and proportionate quantities and along with proper running and sweatout.

Its effects can be quite dramatic so one should understand what niacin is and does before starting the Purification program.

Niacin Research and Radiation

I conducted some research using niacin in 1950. At that

1. **niacin:** a white, odorless, crystalline substance found in protein foods or prepared synthetically. It is a member of the vitamin B complex. *See also* **vitamin B complex**.

2. **Vitamin B complex:** an important group of water-soluble vitamins found in liver, yeast, etc., including vitamin B_1, vitamin B_2 and niacin.

time we referred to niacin as nicotinic acid and the beginning dosage used was 200 mg. (milligrams).

This research was very interesting. Odd manifestations occurred when this vitamin was administered to individuals. Its most startling effect was that it would turn on, in a red flush,[3] a sunburn on the person's body in an exact pattern of a bathing suit! These were very neat patterns. The bathing suit outline was unmistakable.

What kind of "educated vitamin" was this that caused bodies to turn on a flush exactly like a previous sunburn, showing the exact pattern of a bathing suit outline? And which left on the body a pattern of an unaffected area which had been covered by a bathing suit some years before?

Strangely, both the British and American pharmacopoeias[4] advertised that this substance, nicotinic acid (niacin), turned on a flush and was therefore toxic in overdoses.

What we found in 1950 was that if the niacin was continued—in what the pharmacopoeia would term "overdoses"—eventually one got no more flushes from it.

The sunburnlike flushes would eventually disappear at 200 mg., then at 500 mg. they would recur but with less intensity. One might get a small reaction then at 1000 mg. for several days, after which one might administer 2000 mg. and find no more effects. The person would feel fine, his "sunburn" would

3. **flush:** the reddening of the skin caused by a rush of blood; also, the rush of blood itself.

4. **pharmacopoeias:** authoritative books containing lists and descriptions of drugs and medicinal products together with the standards established under law for their production, dispensation, use, etc.

be gone, and he would experience no more flush from the niacin.

But if niacin was toxic, how was it that the more you "overdosed" it the sooner you no longer experienced the sunburnlike flushes from it?

Niacin Reaction—1956

In 1956 I put this vitamin to use again.

At that time there was a lot of bomb testing going on and general radiation exposure. We were working with individuals who had been subjected to atomic tests, atomic accidents and, in at least one case, to materials that had been part of an old atomic explosion. We were engaged in salvaging these people, handling the mental image pictures, stress and upset attendant on these experiences and we succeeded.

But in 1956 niacin was reacting differently on people than it had in 1950, and the effects were more severe.

People on the research program in 1950 had experienced only past sunburn flushes. In 1956 people on the research program, while experiencing a flush, were also experiencing nausea, skin irritations, hives,[5] colitis[6] and other uncomfortable manifestations, on the same vitamin and in the same dosages as had been used in 1950.

The vitamin formula in use *minus* the niacin did not

---

5. **hives:** a disease in which the skin itches and shows raised, white welts, caused by a sensitivity to certain foods or a reaction to heat, light, etc.

6. **colitis:** inflammation of the colon (a part of the large intestine).

---

produce the same effect. Therefore it was obvious that it was the niacin causing these interesting manifestations.

What was this?

The behavior of niacin had been studied in 1950. In regard to sunburnlike flushes we knew what it would do—continued long enough the sunburnlike flushes seemed to discharge.

Why, in 1956, was it producing a different manifestation? The niacin or nicotinic acid hadn't changed. The bodies we were testing hadn't changed. We even tested some of the same people who had been on the research program in 1950, and they now had a different reaction to niacin. What about a case that had had all the sunburn discharged by niacin in 1950 who now, given niacin in 1956, was turning on other sorts of things? Isn't it interesting that just six years later the same vitamin, niacin, was producing an entirely different manifestation?

The *similarity* was that, with the dosages continued long enough, these new manifestations also discharged and disappeared.

The writers of the pharmacopoeia or the biochemist may continue to think that niacin turns on a flush and that it will always turn on a flush in "overdoses."

But the interesting part of it is that it comes to a point where it doesn't turn on a flush. This doesn't happen by conditioning of the body; that is not what occurs. It runs something out.[7]

What does it run out? We knew, from 1950, that it ran out

---

7. **runs out:** erases; causes to disappear.

sunburn, which is a radiation burn. And in 1956 the symptoms those on the research program were experiencing—the nausea, vomiting, skin irritations, colitis and nasal disturbances which accompany radiation sickness—were also discharging with the administration of niacin.

Niacin in 1956 was no longer just running out sunburn. It was running out something which exactly paralleled radiation sickness.

Niacin, then, apparently seems to have a catalytic[8] effect on running out radiation exposure. It seems to give it a kick and run it through.

It will often cause a very hot flush and prickly, itchy skin, which can last up to an hour or longer. It may also bring on chills or make one feel tired.

Medical thinking has been that niacin itself turned on a flush. Something called "niacinamide" was then invented to keep from turning on this flush. Niacin all by itself does not turn on any flush. What it starts to do is immediately run out sunburn or radiation. So the niacinamide that was invented to prevent this flush is worthless (at least for use on the Purification program).

On the Purification program, because quantities of niacin are taken and because of the heat of the sauna, it is possible that it can have the effect of discharging a certain amount, possibly not all, of the accumulated radiation in people.*

* For more information on radiation, read the book *All About Radiation* by L. Ron Hubbard.

8. **catalytic:** causing or accelerating a chemical change without itself (the substance causing the change) being affected.

Unleashing Drugs and Toxins

Taken in sufficient quantities niacin appears to break up and unleash LSD, marijuana and other drugs and poisons from the tissues and cells. It can rapidly release LSD crystals into the system and send a person who has taken LSD on a "trip." (One fellow who had done the earlier Sweat Program for a period of months, and who believed he had no more LSD in his system, took 100 milligrams of niacin and promptly turned on a restimulation of a full-blown LSD experience.)

Running and sweating must be done in conjunction with taking niacin to ensure the toxic substances it releases actually do get flushed out of the body.

Recently, doctors in megavitamin research have been administering niacin to get people through withdrawal symptoms or get them over bad drug kicks. They have been using enormous doses of, for example, 5000 mg. of niacin.

I have no personal knowledge that such enormous doses are necessary for handling drugs, though they well may be in some cases. It is very possible that, given the combination of all the points on the Purification program, many people would be able to handle drugs with lesser amounts of niacin, something under 5000 mg.

Niacin Theory: Running through Past Deficiencies

In theory, niacin apparently does not do anything by itself. It is simply interacting with niacin deficiencies which already exist in the cellular structure. It doesn't turn on allergies; it appears to run out allergies. Evidently anything that niacin does is the result of running out and running through past deficiencies.

Caution: The manifestations niacin produces can be quite horrifying. Some of the somatics[9] and manifestations the person may turn on are not just somatics in lots of cases, in my experience. For example, I have seen a full-blown case of skin cancer turn on and run out on niacin dosages. So it appears that a person can turn on skin cancer with this and, if that should happen, the handling, by observable fact, has been to continue the niacin until the skin cancer has run out completely.

Other lesser manifestations that may turn on with niacin are hives, flu symptoms, gastroenteritis,[10] aching bones, upset stomach or a fearful or terrified condition. There seems to be no limit to the variety of phenomena that may occur with niacin. If the deficiency is there to be turned on by niacin it apparently will do so with niacin.

The two vital facts here, proven by observation, are:

1. When the niacin was carried on until these things discharged they did then vanish, as they *will* do. Sometimes people get timid about it and don't finish the program, which leaves them hung up in a deficiency that is creating a particular illness or manifestation. This should not be allowed to happen.

    It is a matter of record that a reaction turned on by niacin will turn off where administration of niacin is continued.

---

9. **somatics:** physical pains or discomforts of any kind. The word *somatic* means, actually, bodily or physical. Because the word *pain* has in the past led to confusion between physical pain and mental pain, *somatic* is the term used to denote physical pain or discomfort.

10. **gastroenteritis:** an inflammation of the stomach and the intestines.

2. When the niacin dosage was increased and the whole lot of the rest of the vitamins being taken was also increased proportionately, the niacin itself, taken in large amounts, did not create a vitamin deficiency.

Created Nutritional Failure

On the Purification program it is the progressive increase of the niacin dosages that determines the proportionate increase of the other vitamins and minerals.

Thus, what could slow down the Purification program and make it appear incomplete would be a nutritional failure—a failure to flank the niacin on either side by sufficient amounts of the other needed vitamins and minerals in proportion and a failure to provide food intake which included vegetables (with their vitamin and mineral content) and oil.

In such a case one would be looking at created nutritional deficiencies—not conditions which were there, necessarily, at the outset of the program.

Not knowing these things is possibly what made medics earlier believe that niacin itself had side effects. The side effects were probably somatics and manifestations of already existing deficiencies only half run out and deficiencies created by not flanking niacin with the other vitamins and minerals and oils necessary to permit a rebuild.

10

Nutrition and Deficiencies

10

Nutrition and Deficiencies

Many people probably begin taking drugs because they feel terrible due to dietary deficiencies. These then progressively worsen, as the drugs *themselves* cause wholesale[1] vitamin and mineral deficiencies. Recovery from drugs requires a full repair of these deficiencies.

Having been an early discoverer and instigator of vitamin therapy I know whereof I speak on the subject of nutritional deficiencies. Some of my work covering vitamins and deficiencies, stimulants and depressants and the field of biochemistry, goes back to the spring of 1950 and earlier. Studies made in those fields were highly contributive to evolving the Purification program.

Minerals: Key to Glandular Interaction

Between 1945 and 1973 I studied the endocrine system.[2] From this study it seemed apparent that minerals and trace

---

1. **wholesale:** extensive; broadly indiscriminate.

2. **endocrine system:** the system of glands which produce one or more internal secretions that, introduced directly into the bloodstream, are carried to other parts of the body whose functions they regulate or control.

---

minerals[3] operating in the bloodstream and circulated by other body fluids were a key to glandular interaction.

The theory is: Every gland in the body specializes in one or more minerals and, actually, that is how the glands make themselves interact with one another. In other words, the endocrine system of the body monitors itself apparently through minerals.

As various drugs upset the whole endocrine system, one can see that the moment one starts administering vitamins and extensive sweating and such actions, one is going to get a mineral demand in the body. Therefore, there would need to be certain mineral dosages right along with the rest of this package.

When one is conversant with the subject of nutrition and with the elements of the program, it is obvious that in the face of an unhandled vitamin or mineral deficiency the effectiveness of the procedure will suffer.

Thus, nutrition and nutritional deficiencies are both vital topics for discussion in any text on this program.

Drugs and Toxins Cause Vitamin Burn-up

One of the things that toxins and drugs do is create nutritional deficiencies in the body in the form of vitamin and mineral deficiencies. A vitamin C[4] deficiency, a B_1 deficiency, a

---

3. **trace minerals:** minerals that are required in minute quantities for physiological functioning.

4. **vitamin C:** also called ascorbic acid; a colorless, crystalline, water-soluble vitamin, found in many foods, especially citrus fruits, vegetables and rose hips and also made synthetically; it is required for proper nutrition and metabolism.

B complex deficiency and a niacin deficiency are brought about by drugs. There may be other deficiencies caused by drugs that we are not aware of at this time. But that list is certain.

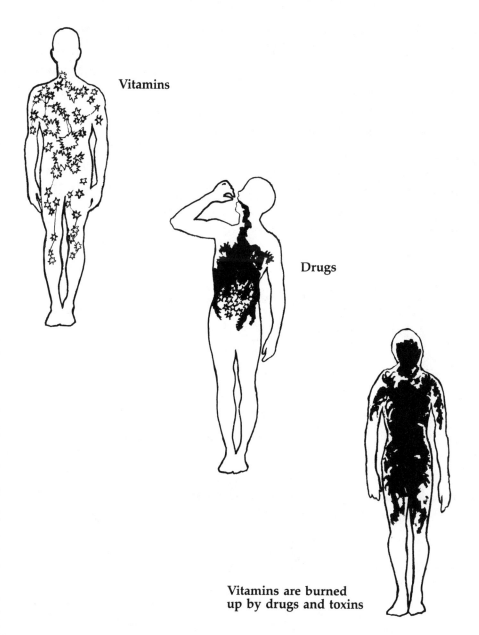

Vitamins

Drugs

Vitamins are burned up by drugs and toxins

Also, alcohol, for example, depends for its effects upon the body being able to burn up B_1. When it burns up all the B_1 in the system the person goes into delirium tremens[5] and nightmares.

In the case of other toxic substances, the probability exists that other vitamins are burned up. What we seem to have hit upon here is that LSD and other street drugs burn up not only B_1 and B complex but also create a deficiency of niacin in the body and that they possibly depend on niacin, one of the B complex vitamins, for their effect.

In light of the discovery that toxic and drug residuals can remain in the body for years, it can be assumed that these residuals, to the degree that they are still present, might have the same and continuing effect on the body's reserves of vitamins and minerals.

Deficiencies and Illness

Any vital substances on which body support depends, when too reduced or omitted from consumption, can be depended upon to result in a nonoptimum physical condition.

When very obvious, it becomes a "disease." And when less obvious and even undetected, it becomes a "not feeling good."

There is a distinct possibility that (after mental and spiritual factors) the largest contributive factor in aging is the composite of cumulative deficiencies.

---

5. **delirium tremens:** a violent delirium (temporary state of extreme mental excitement, marked by restlessness, confused speech and hallucinations) resulting chiefly from excessive drinking of alcoholic liquor and characterized by sweating, trembling, anxiety and frightening hallucinations. *Delirium tremens* comes from Latin, and means literally "trembling delirium."

Predisposition[6] to other types of illness is in many instances occasioned by these deficiencies even when the precipitation[7] is viral[8] or bacterial.[9]

Prolongation of illness is guaranteed when deficiencies remain present and unremedied.

Thus, a factor in the development of the Purification program was to handle any such deficiency with sufficient daily quantities of vitamins and minerals in addition to whatever was supplied the person through his regular meals.

The exact quantities of the substances used on the program are given in the next chapter of this book. As a part of the program itself, these then would be increased proportionately according to individual need.

Artificial Deficiencies

A vitamin or mineral does not work alone—it must be accompanied by other elements with which it combines to do its work.

---

6. **predisposition:** the fact or condition of having an inclination or tendency to beforehand; susceptibility.

7. **precipitation:** a being caused to happen before expected, warranted, needed or desired; a bringing on; a hastening.

8. **viral:** of or caused by a *virus:* a form of matter smaller than any of the bacteria, that can multiply in living cells and cause disease in animals or plants (smallpox, measles, the flu, etc., are caused by viruses).

9. **bacterial:** caused by *bacteria,* typically one-celled organisms which can be seen only with a microscope. They occur in three main forms—spherical, rod-shaped and spiral; some bacteria cause diseases such as pneumonia and tuberculosis, and others are necessary for fermentation, decomposition, etc.

For example, when one gives B_6,[10] a complimentary amount of B_2[11] has to be given for it to be effective. It is all very well to say that B_6 helps the nervous system and without it all sorts of things happen. But should one start giving a fellow B_6 and then wonder why nothing spectacular occurs, it is because he isn't also being given a complimentary quantity of B_2.

When large dosages of certain vitamins, minerals or food-stuffs are given, an artificial deficiency can apparently be created of others not given. Increases in some elements, just by the fact of their being increased, demand increases in others. When intake of some elements is markedly increased, *balance* must be maintained by proportionately increasing others.

Lacking needed elements in one area, the body will even rob bones, muscles and tissue to obtain the missing elements.

Artificial deficiencies can be so created.

This is a principle I hit upon as early as 1950 and proved it. You can actually create a deficiency in C by administering B and calcium. All you have to do is pump those things to a fellow in very, very heavy dosages and he will develop the characteristics of C deficiency. His teeth begin to hurt. Then, when you give him C, the manifestations go away. In other words, an overdose of "X" and "Y" can apparently create a deficiency in "Z."

The reason for this is that a vitamin is making certain changes in the body and these changes, to occur fully, also

---

10. **B_6:** a vitamin, also called pyridoxine, important as an enzyme activator in protein, carbohydrate and fat metabolism, hormone production (adrenalin and insulin) and antibody production.

11. **B_2:** also called riboflavin, a vitamin important in the metabolism of protein and in skin, liver and eye health.

require the additional vitamin. But if that additional vitamin isn't there, it gives the manifestation of being in deficiency.

The principle here is that by giving one or two vitamins in excess amount you can create a nutritional deficiency of another vitamin which isn't being given or isn't being given in enough quantity. This would apply to minerals as well.

Thus, vitamin and mineral rations would have to be taken in proportion to one another.

This theory was a major element in the development of the Purification program and remains a major element in its successful and effective delivery.

11

Nutritional Supplements

11

Nutritional Supplements

To repeat the point made in an earlier chapter, special diets and food fads are no part of this program.

What *is* part of this scene is that the person will need certain nutrition in the form of vitamins and minerals in addition to his regular meals. One follows his normal eating habits; there are no *deletions* of certain foods required. There are, however, some *additions* to the normal eating habits. These consist of, in addition to the person's regular meals:

a. Plenty of vegetables which have not been over-cooked. Vegetables contain a lot of minerals and fiber as well as specific important vitamins.

b. A quantity of the recommended oil—ensuring that it is fresh—taken daily. (This would be an oil combining the four oils: soy, peanut, walnut and safflower oil, plus lecithin.)

c. Vitamin and mineral supplements in the exact dosages recommended, increased proportionately as the program progresses.

d. One to three glasses of "Cal-Mag" (the calcium-magnesium drink), daily, as advised.

e. Plenty of water and other liquids taken daily, to help flush out the system.

Vitamins and Minerals

As a record of research, listed below are the approximate daily amounts of the various vitamins and minerals taken by most persons when starting the program. It is important that no one of these vitamins or minerals is taken to the exclusion of another or others.

Niacin:	100 mg. (or less, depending upon individual tolerance at the start) daily.
Vitamin B complex:	approximately 2 tablets daily, each tablet containing the same amounts of B_2 and B_6.
Vitamin B_1:	250–500 mg. daily, in addition to the B_1 contained in the B complex tablet.
Vitamin A:	approximately 5000 IU[1] daily.
Vitamin D:	approximately 400 IU daily. (This is usually taken in a capsule that is a combination of 400 IU of vitamin D and the 5000 IU of vitamin A listed above.)
Vitamin C:	approximately 250–1000 mg. daily, depending upon individual tolerance.
Vitamin E:	approximately 800 IU daily.
Multi-Minerals:	1 to 2 tablets daily, each containing a balanced combination of minerals.
"Cal-Mag" Formula:	at least one glass, or more as advised, daily. (The "Cal-Mag" Formula, described in Chapter 9, Part 1 of this book,

1. **IU:** abbreviation for *international unit*, an internationally agreed-upon standard to which samples of a substance, as a drug or hormone, are compared to ascertain their relative potency. *IU* also stands for the particular quantity of such a substance which causes a specific biological effect.

provides extra quantities of the minerals calcium and magnesium, and this is taken daily in addition to the daily multi-mineral tablets.)

Vitamin B Complex

The vitamin B complex tablet that was used in the initial research for the Purification program was one which contained:

B_1:	50 mg.	Folic Acid:[2]	100 mcg.
B_2:	50 mg.	Biotin:[3]	50 mcg.
B_6:	50 mg.	Choline:[4]	50 mg.
B_{12}:[5]	50 mcg.	Niacinamide:	50 mg.
Pantothenic Acid:[6]	50 mg.	Inositol:[7]	50 mg.
PABA:[8]	50 mg.		

all in a base of lecithin, parsley, rice bran, watercress and alfalfa.

The same tablet or one with similar content is still used very successfully in delivering the Purification program.

2. **folic acid:** a vitamin important in the formation of red blood cells.

3. **biotin:** a vitamin important in protein, carbohydrate and unsaturated fatty acid metabolism, normal growth and maintenance of skin, hair, nerves, bone marrow and various glands.

4. **choline:** a vitamin important to the functioning of the nervous system (it is an essential ingredient in the nerve fluid), the liver and the buildup of immunities.

5. **B_{12}:** a vitamin important to red blood cell formation, nervous system health, normal growth, carbohydrate metabolism and fertility.

6. **pantothenic acid:** an acid found in plant and animal tissues, rice, bran, etc., that is part of the B complex of vitamins and is essential for cell growth.

7. **inositol:** a vitamin found in high concentrations in the human brain, stomach, kidney, spleen and liver; related to control of cholesterol level; reported to have mild inhibitory effect on cancer.

8. **PABA:** an abbreviation for a vitamin called *para-amino-benzoic* acid; important in the metabolism of protein, blood cell formation, stimulation of intestinal bacteria to produce folic acid and utilization of pantothenic acid. *See also* **folic acid** and **pantothenic acid.**

Mineral Tablet

The multi-mineral tablet used in the initial research was one containing the following mineral amounts per each nine tablets. In other words, one tablet would provide *only ⅑ of the following mineral amounts:*

500 mg. calcium	4 mg. manganese[9]
250 mg. magnesium	2 mg. copper
18 mg. iron	45 mg. potassium (protein complex)
15 mg. zinc	.225 mg. iodine[10] (kelp).

In the tablet used, the minerals (with the exception of the potassium and the iodine) are "chelated"[11] (bonded with) amino acids[12] in a base of selenium,[13] yeast, DNA,[14] RNA,[15] ginseng,[16] alfalfa leaf flour, parsley, watercress and cabbage.

---

9. **manganese:** a mineral important to growth, bone formation, reproduction, muscle coordination and fat and carbohydrate metabolism.

10. **iodine:** a chemical element found in seawater and certain seaweeds, used in solution as an antiseptic; iodine is used by the thyroid gland (a large gland at the front of the neck, secreting a hormone that regulates the body's growth and development) to help regulate metabolism, and a shortage of iodine can cause goiter (enlargement of the thyroid gland).

11. **chelated:** a process by which minerals are held, as if by a claw, by amino acids. *Chelation* is taken from a Greek word meaning "claw." This bonding of a mineral with an amino acid exists in nature as a necessary step for the mineral to be absorbed and used by the body. Thus, with this step already provided, the mineral is more easily absorbed and used. *See also* **amino acids**.

12. **amino acids:** basic organic compounds which are essential to the body's breakdown and absorption of foods.

13. **selenium:** a trace mineral which helps to keep muscles healthy, protect cells against oxidation and stimulate the manufacture of antibodies.

The same mineral tablet, or one with similar content or additional minerals, is still used effectively on the program.

High Mineral Dosages

Initially, on the program, mineral dosages were started at one to two tablets daily. Then, as the niacin and other vitamins were increased in proportion to each other, the mineral dosages were increased accordingly in increments of two to three tablets, three to four tablets, four to five tablets and five to six tablets taken daily.

Later research then indicated that much higher mineral dosages than these gave most optimum results on the program. (See Mineral Table on page 124.)

Large amounts of minerals are lost in sweating in the sauna. Thus, high, high quantities of minerals must be taken to replenish those flushed out by sweating.

Additionally, it is possible that as an individual progresses on the program there is often an improvement in the ability of the body to assimilate the minerals it needs.

---

14. **DNA:** abbreviation for *deoxyribonucleic acid*; a complex compound found in the nucleus of all living cells which plays a vital part in heredity. It is the chief material in chromosomes, the cell bodies that control the heredity of an animal or a plant. The DNA in the chromosomes furnishes the cells with a complete set of "instructions" for their own development and the development of their descendants for generations.

15. **RNA:** abbreviation for *ribonucleic acid*; one of the compounds found in all living cells; the substance that carries out DNA's instructions for protein production. *See also* **DNA.**

16. **ginseng:** any of several plants of eastern Asia or North America having an aromatic root used medicinally.

Proportionate Vitamin/Mineral Increases

The tables on the next pages provide the data on how the vitamins and minerals should be increased, in ratio, as the person progresses on the program.

It is the gradient increase of niacin which monitors the gradient increase of the other vitamins and minerals given on the program. The niacin is increased correspondingly with the decrease of reaction from the niacin, as covered fully in the next chapter. Vitamins B_1 and C particularly have to keep pace with the niacin as it is increased in dosage, in order to prevent creating artificial vitamin deficiencies.

The dosages in these tables show the variations of individual tolerances encountered and the ranges of increase which have proven most effective in the majority of cases.

(see tables on following pages)

Vitamin Table

This table shows proportionate vitamin increases at various stages of the program.

	Stage 1	Stage 2	Stage 3	Stage 4	Stage 5
Niacin	100 to 400 mg.	500 to 1400 mg.	1500 to 2400 mg.	2500 to 3400 mg.	3500 to 5000 mg.
Vitamin A	5000 to 10,000 IU	20,000 IU	30,000 IU	50,000 IU	50,000 IU
Vitamin D	400 IU	800 IU	1200 IU	2000 IU	2000 IU
Vitamin C	250 to 1000 mg.	2 to 3 gm.	3 to 4 gm.	4 to 5 gm.	5 to 6 gm.
Vitamin E	800 IU	1200 IU	1600 IU	2000 IU	2400 IU
Vitamin B complex	2 tablets	3 tablets	4 tablets	5 tablets	6 tablets
Vitamin B_1	350 to 600 mg.	400 to 650 mg.	450 to 700 mg.	750 to 1250 mg.	800 to 1300 mg.

Mineral Table

The following table shows the approximate mineral amounts now found to give best results at the various stages of vitamin increase.

	Stage 1	Stage 2	Stage 3	Stage 4	Stage 5
(All figures in milligrams except those for Cal-Mag)					
Calcium	500 to 1000	1000 to 1500	1500 to 2000	2000 to 2500	2500 to 3000
Magnesium	250 to 500	500 to 750	750 to 1000	1000 to 1250	1250 to 1500
Iron	18–36	36–54	54–72	72–90	90–108
Zinc	15–30	30–45	45–60	60–75	75–90
Manganese	4–8	8–12	12–16	16–20	20–24
Copper	2–4	4–6	6–8	8–10	10–12
Potassium	45–90	90–135	135–180	180–225	225–270
Iodine	.225 to .450	.450 to .675	.675 to .900	.900 to 1.125	1.125 to 1.350
Cal-Mag	1 – 1½ glasses	1 – 2 glasses	1 – 2 glasses	2 – 3 glasses	2 – 3 glasses

(Note: The number of mineral tablets to be taken would depend upon the strength of the particular tablet used. The importance is that one gets the necessary amounts of the minerals. It has been found that large tablets may not be as easily broken down and absorbed into the body as smaller tablets may be. Thus one might not get the same amount of minerals from a large tablet as from several smaller tablets, even though the large tablet might contain the same amount of minerals.)

How to Read the Tables

As a clarification, first of all, the figures on these tables designating points of increase (Stages 1, 2, 3, 4 and 5) do *not* refer to the first, second, third, fourth and fifth days of the program. They refer to approximate "stages" of vitamin and mineral increase (in relation to the niacin increase) that an individual goes through on the program.

On the Vitamin Table, under Stage 1, the first figure given for each vitamin shows the usual starting dosage of that vitamin used for most individuals. The range then shown under Stage 1 indicates how these starting dosages may be increased within a few days or within a week or so, depending upon the niacin reaction the person is experiencing.

On the Mineral Table, under Stage 1, the first column of figures (reading downward) gives the usual starting mineral dosages for most individuals. The range under Stage 1 shows the possible rate of mineral increase during this first phase of the program.

The same applies to the increments shown at Stages 2, 3, 4 and 5 on both tables.

Example: Person A starts the program on 100 milligrams of niacin plus the other beginning increments of vitamins, per the Vitamin Table. His beginning increments of minerals, per the Mineral Table, are approximately: calcium 500 mg.; magnesium 250 mg.; iron 18 mg.; zinc 15 mg.; manganese 4 mg.; copper 2 mg.; potassium 45 mg.; and iodine .225 mg.

He continues with these daily dosages until the niacin

effects have diminished—in his case this occurs on, let us say, the third day of the program. At that point his niacin dosage is increased to 200 mg. daily, with the other daily vitamins and minerals increased proportionately, and he continues on those dosages until the niacin effects have diminished. Progressing in this way, by the seventh day of the program his vitamin and mineral dosages have been increased up to the levels given in Stage 2 of the tables. After the ninth day his vitamins and minerals may have been increased all the way up to Stage 3 as shown on the tables. And he continues in this way all the way up through the levels of dosages at Stage 5.

This varies from one individual to the next.

Person B, for example, starts on 100 mg. of niacin and the accompanying vitamin and mineral dosages, and may then require a week or more to work up to the levels of vitamin and mineral dosages shown at Stage 2. He may then move rapidly through Stage 2, take another week to move through Stage 3 and actually complete the program at some point on Stage 4.

There is no rote pattern to be followed. It is totally a matter of standardly applying the data given as to when the niacin should be increased. (See Part One, Chapter 12, "Increasing the Niacin.") That is the factor that may vary widely from one individual to the next.

However, the tables given on the previous pages show the guidelines which were and are still followed for increasing the vitamin and mineral increments proportionately at the times the niacin is increased.

Additional Notes on Vitamins

It should be stressed here that individual tolerances were and always must be taken into consideration in each case.

Quantities of vitamin C especially would need to be carefully increased according to the person's tolerance of it, as too much vitamin C can result in stomach upsets or diarrhea for some people.

At the same time, it is important that the vitamin C increase keeps pace, proportionately, with the niacin increase. Records exist where vitamin C has become so deficient in a drug user that he could use up tens of thousands of milligrams of C per day before he begins to eliminate any. A severe vitamin C deficiency can result in the disease called scurvy.[17] "Live C" from raw onions or raw potatoes is sometimes necessary in addition to synthetic vitamin C. (These were the traditional remedies for scurvy.)

Vitamins and minerals should *not* be taken on an empty stomach, as they could cause stomach burn. They should be taken after meals or, if taken between meals, with yogurt.

Niacinamide

The majority of vitamin B complex tablets on the market include niacinamide in small amounts. This is the substance invented by someone to keep an individual from turning on a niacin flush. Because it does prevent a niacin flush, niacinamide is worthless.

---

17. **scurvy:** a disease resulting from a deficiency of ascorbic acid (vitamin C) in the body, characterized by weakness, anemia, spongy gums, bleeding from the mucous membranes, etc.

The likelihood is that the amount of niacinamide in a B complex tablet acts only to eliminate any flush from the niacin content in that specific tablet. Results from the piloting of the Purification program, where plenty of niacin flush was experienced on different dosages of niacin itself (in combination with the flanking vitamins and minerals), indicate that the inclusion of niacinamide in the B complex had little if any effect upon the flush that resulted from the additional dosages of niacin taken. However, where a B complex tablet can be found that includes niacin rather than niacinamide, that would be the preferable tablet to use.

It is also possible to have a B complex tablet especially made up that includes actual niacin *instead of* niacinamide, in amounts equal to the B_1, B_2 and B_6 amounts, particularly if one is ordering the tablet in fairly large amounts.

Note: Where a B complex tablet that includes niacin is used, this adds that much more to the daily niacin intake and this must be taken into consideration when increasing niacin and B complex dosages.

Additional Notes on Minerals: Trace Minerals

Most multiple mineral formulas include the major mineral elements required by the body but not all of the trace minerals.

"Trace" minerals are those minerals which have been found essential to maintaining life, even though they are found in the body in very small, i.e., "trace" amounts.

The main trace minerals currently include: cobalt, copper, iodine, manganese, molybdenum, zinc, selenium and chromium. Tin was also added as an essential trace mineral as late as 1970.

Nutritional researchists are the first to admit that the work in this field is very far from complete, and there will undoubtedly be other trace minerals added to the list as such research is continued.

Currently, also, there are fairly wide differences of opinion among nutritionists as to the minimum daily requirements of the various minerals and especially the trace minerals.

Minerals are found in a wide variety of foods. Natural foods, undamaged by processing, are the best sources of minerals as they exist in unprocessed foods in the combinations in which they are most effective. But minerals can also be lacking in foods grown in mineral-depleted soil. Additionally, of course, there is no one food that supplies them all.

Therefore, it may be necessary to use more than one type of multi-mineral tablet to ensure one is getting all of the minerals, including the trace minerals, that are required by the body.

Note: The Vitamin and Mineral Tables given on the preceding pages do not include any additional vitamins or minerals which might be needed in cases of specific deficiencies an individual might have. Any such particular deficiency would need to be determined by a medical doctor and remedied with the additional vitamin or mineral dosages recommended.

As a guideline, four of the more informative books on the subject of nutritional vitamins and minerals are the following by Adelle Davis: *Let's Get Well, Let's Eat Right to Keep Fit, Let's Cook It Right* and *Let's Have Healthy Children.*

The research data offered in this chapter is not to be

construed as a recommendation of medical treatment or medication. It is given here as a record of food supplements in the form of the nutritional vitamins and minerals which were used in the development of the Purification program and which were found to be most effective in the greatest number of cases.

12

Increasing
the Niacin

12

Increasing the Niacin

Increasing Niacin and Other Vitamin Quantities

Most persons who have done the Purification program started at 100 mg. of niacin (some took lesser amounts at the start, depending upon tolerance) and increased the dosage as they progressed.

The best results were obtained when niacin was taken all at one time, not split up during the day. Taken with water on an empty stomach it can be very upsetting. It is found to be best taken after a meal, or with yogurt or milk.

To increase the dosage, a specific quantity of niacin was administered each day until the effect that dosage produced diminished. One would then, next day, up the dosage on a gradient, say, in amounts of 100 mg. In this way you get an overlap of the old dosage becoming useless and the new dosage being needed. This tended to speed up the action considerably when continued each time the effect of the dosage diminished.

The other vitamins would have to be increased proportionately to niacin at the same time the niacin is increased, as they are interacting in the deficiencies and more are needed.

It was found essential that C, B_1 and other B vitamins need to be given in ratio to the niacin being fed. In other words, as you up the niacin you would up the B_1 and the B complex. And also as niacin is upped, the vitamin C would be upped. These things would have to be kept in ratio.

How and When to Increase the Niacin

Within the boundaries of the medical doctor's advice for the individual, the most workable gradient in the majority of cases observed was generally found to be starting the person on 100 mg. of niacin and increasing it in increments of 100 mg. until the person was up to 1000 mg. daily. A steeper gradient was then used as one went up to higher dosages. It was found that many persons could take increases of from 300 to 500 mg. at one time when they reached the higher dosage ranges. Note that this does not refer to a *daily* increase, necessarily, but refers to the gradient in which the dosage was upped when an increased dosage was indicated.

Any increase was always based on individual tolerance and there were exceptions to the "generally successful gradient" described above. Certain individuals would and did require moving up on a lesser gradient according to their tolerances and according to medical advices.

On the other hand, a "grinding" phenomenon was observed where the individual:

    a. held to a certain niacin dosage of, say, 500 mg. day after day, until nothing whatsoever was happening

or

    b. held to an increase of only 100 mg. at a time in the

higher ranges of niacin, even though he was getting only brief, mild results, was very able to tolerate these effects and felt he could handle a steeper gradient.

By "grinding" phenomenon is meant an effect similar to doing something over and over with the person becoming irritated and frustrated with the program and feeling he is not making the progress he could be making.

In these instances, it was observed that when the persons who could progress at a faster rate with larger niacin increases (always with the other vitamins and minerals increased in the correct ratio and by individual tolerance) did so, they went smoothly along on the program handling what did crop up.

When to introduce an increase in niacin was found to be as important as the amount of increase.

When niacin was increased:

a. after the effect of a certain dosage had *diminished* (not vanished totally)

and

b. when any *other* manifestations and restimulation which had turned on at that dosage had diminished or totally disappeared (as covered earlier in the stated procedure), good progress was made on the program on a one for one basis, providing all other points of the program were standardly being applied.

In other words, it was recognized that there would very likely be various reactions and restimulations (as covered earlier), all of which would need to be taken into consideration when niacin amounts were increased.

When this was done correctly, excellent results were obtained. Questions arising on such increases were handled according to the person's individual medical approval to do the program and further medical advices as needed.

Caution

It should be mentioned here that, along with this research data, reports have been received of persons found taking niacin quietly on their own without being on the Purification program and without being under any supervision, medical or otherwise, just to see what it would handle. This is not advised. It could result in artificially created deficiencies or in things turning on which are not then properly handled or resolved.

Powder Versus Tablet

Some persons have reported more immediate and/or intense results when niacin was taken in powder form. This difference was most often reported by persons who had reached the higher dosages, had little or no results from a large, highly compressed tablet, and then switched to the same dosage in powder form and got more intense results.

However, several people report that they got results when taking 100, 200, 300 and 400 mg. of niacin in tablets of 100 mg. each; then, when 500 mg. were taken in a single 500 mg. tablet, nothing occurred. However, the next day, when 500 mg. were taken in 5 tablets of 100 mg. each, results were obtained at the 500 mg. dosage.

Still others reported effective results from niacin tablets of any dosage, including the larger tablets of higher dosage.

What has been done effectively is to use tablets of 100 mg. niacin each until the 1000 mg. niacin dosage is reached and to use niacin in powder form thereafter. Where this is done, or where niacin in powder form is used exclusively, the measurement must be exactly done.

The label on a powdered niacin container should carry instructions as to how to measure the powder content. With the brands that have been used, 1 teaspoon provides 3,000 mg. of pure niacin. *Note:* This is per the English system of weights and measures. One would need to use the standard measuring teaspoon. In areas of the world where the metric system is used (and where "teaspoon" sizes vary), an amount equivalent to a standard teaspoon measurement would be 4.9 milliliters.

13

The End Phenomena of the Purification Program

13

The End Phenomena of the Purification Program

What Is Meant by "End Phenomena"?

The end phenomena of any action could be said to be those indicators which are present when the action has been fully and correctly completed.

The purpose of the Purification program is very simply to clean out and purify one's system of all the accumulated impurities such as drugs and other toxic chemical substances, e.g., food preservatives, insecticides, pesticides, etc. For someone who has taken LSD or angel dust this would include getting rid of any residual crystals from the body.

The end phenomena is reached when the individual is free of the restimulative presence of residuals of past chemicals, drugs and other toxic substances. He will no longer be feeling the effects of these impurities going into restimulation and there is usually a marked resurgence of overall sense of well-being.

Niacin Dosages at Completion

Per research data, there are a number of people who have completed the program to full end phenomena on dosages under 5000 mg. of niacin. Others have gone as high as that dosage before completing.

There is no hard and fast rule laid down anywhere that says a person must work up to 5000 mg. of niacin before he is complete.

How to Recognize Valid End Phenomena

As the person goes through the Purification program, one should be able to see an improvement in both his physical well-being and general outlook on life as he rids the system of its accumulated toxins.

Obviously if the person is still feeling the effects of past drugs or chemicals going into restimulation, the program cannot be considered complete and must be continued until all such manifestations have turned off completely.

Per research data collected, where a person was progressing well on the program one could observe him becoming more mentally alert and aware. He would start reporting exactly what was going on, what substance was turning on, what impurities and restimulations he was running out. He could usually tell if he had hit a tolerance level on a certain vitamin. All of these are valid reactions throughout the program.

As the person would run out whatever was there to turn on, the manifestations became less day by day, and he would reach a point where no further manifestations were coming up. He would look and feel remarkably better, brighter and more alert; he would have come through with good wins[1] and he

---

1. **wins:** gains or realizations. Also, intending to do something and doing it or intending not to do something and not doing it. For example, if one intends to be able to communicate better with his boss and does so, that is a win. Or if one intends to no longer be shy around girls and accomplishes that, it is a win.

would often know and state that he felt free of toxic residuals and their associated restimulative effects (though not necessarily in those exact words), and originate on his own that he had completed the program. With all those indicators, one could be pretty sure he *had* completed it.

The amount of vitamins and mineral nutrients, exercise and sweatout it has taken and will take to accomplish this on the Purification program is an individual matter in each case.

Drug History and Completion

The fact of having a heavy drug history does not necessarily prolong the program, although it can do so. More important than anything else is keeping all points of the program in standardly, maintaining a well-balanced personal schedule with enough rest and nutrients, and getting in the prescribed period of exercise and sauna on a routine daily basis.

On such a schedule, persons of varying drug histories, some heavy, some light, have completed the program in eighteen to twenty days at five hours a day, reaching the end phenomena at amounts of niacin (and the flanking vitamin and mineral nutrients) which differed with different individuals. Some have done so in less time, some have taken longer.

Following Program Completion

A continuation of the vitamins, minerals, oil, vegetables and Cal-Mag, at least at the rate of the minimum recommended daily requirements in balanced amounts is wise after the program has been completed. Otherwise, a sudden cessation of such heavy vitamin dosages can produce a letdown.[2] It is possible the person should come off on a steep gradient rather than cease abruptly. Particularly where drug damage to the brain or nerves has occurred, the body needs these things to rebuild itself. If one doesn't continue the essential nutrients there can be the apparency of a letdown.

Remember that the person has probably been leading an unhealthy life without proper nutrition, sleep or exercise. Or, even where he has kept these health factors in, he has been subjected to the pollutants and toxins which surround us daily. Thus, it would be a good idea to recommend moderate daily dietetic and exercise disciplines so he can stay healthy. Such disciplines are not therapy; they are simply a matter of good common sense.

Note that upon completion of the program, it is *not* intended that one gradiently does less of *all* the elements of the Purification program, e.g., less sauna, less exercise, less vitamins, etc., each day, tapering down to cessation of these actions.

The suggestion that *is* made is that one doesn't abruptly simply cease the extra nutrients he has been taking, but comes down from high dosages on a steep gradient to what would be a moderate normal daily requirement for him, per medical advices. And along with this, some moderate daily exercise can help him maintain good health.

Continuing all the elements of the Purification program would amount to continuing the program itself past the point of valid completion, and that is not the intention.

---

2. **letdown:** a decrease in energy, force, volume, etc.

What Comes Next?

Upon completion of the Purification program, the person is now in good shape to receive gains from mental or spiritual improvement programs and get optimum gain from them.

Thus, we are not looking at an endless run on the Purification program. We are seeking simply to handle the drug deposits and toxic residues in their restimulation and reinforcement of mental image pictures and vice versa. And by breaking up the balance of these two and handling the one side of it on the Purification program, we are freeing up the person to be able to handle the other side of it, the mental image picture side of it.

The latter would be accomplished on another and quite different program.

The important thing, however, is that the person is now free to accomplish it, as he is no longer caught up in the constant interaction between the mental recordings of the effects of drugs and toxins, *and* the physical effects of the residual deposits.

Part 2

The Purification Program:

Guidelines for Successful Application

1

Administration of the Purification Program

1

Administration of the Purification Program

The procedure for administration of the Purification program laid out in this chapter is based on the practical experience gained from the research and development of the technology of the program as well as large pilot projects during which it was delivered to some hundreds of individuals. This procedure is geared toward formalized delivery of the Purification program, however it is vital data for the individual doing the program as well. These regulations should not be taken lightly nor disregarded.

Caution

One may find that persons administering the program might tend to enter their own fads or hobbies into it, or, needing it themselves, avoid standard delivery of it.

Examples of this might be: giving advice based only on one's opinion or personal experience which results in alteration of the researched program procedure, hobbyhorsing[1]

---

1. **hobbyhorsing:** concerning oneself excessively with a favorite notion or activity; variation of the phrase *ride a hobbyhorse*.

some particular food fad or diet, injecting personal opinion as to the efficacy of certain vitamins to the exclusion of others, neglecting the importance of maintaining the prescribed schedule and permitting irregularities such as insufficient sleep or insufficient running or sauna time, or advising mixing the Purification program with other procedures.

It is important that those administering the program do so purely and exactly by the regulations governing such administration. If an individual reports difficulties on the program, it is essential to check to see if any such erroneous advice has been tendered[2] by well-meaning friends or by those handling the program in a purely administrative capacity.

Orienting the Participant

To prepare an individual to participate in the Purification program the following steps are taken:

1. Inform the person that he must have medical approval to participate in the program, following a medical exam by an informed and licensed medical practitioner.

2. Brief the person on the basic theory and main elements of the program.

3. Ensure he understands the procedures to be followed, the need for keeping to a routine schedule, getting enough sleep and following the correct vitamin regimen.

4. Ensure he understands that the program does not include medication, and that the vitamins, oils and

2. **tendered:** presented for acceptance; offered.

minerals taken during the program are nutrition, i.e., that they are food, not medicine or drugs.

5. Educate the person on:

   a. the need for taking plenty of liquids to replenish liquids lost during sweating in the sauna and

   b. how to prevent heat exhaustion and how to handle it should it occur.

6. Brief the person on what niacin is, what it does, and what reactions he might experience during the program and why, without making promises as to results.

7. Ensure he understands the importance of continuing the program to its completion, once started on it.

8. Get his promise to follow instructions and complete the program and not abandon it because it becomes uncomfortable or out of laziness or because he/she has other appointments or concerns.

9. Have the person sign a release which covers the above and which clearly states he is undertaking the program on his own volition after having been duly informed as to the purpose and procedure of the program and after having received medical approval to do the program.

Handling any misunderstanding the person may have before he gets started on the program and emphasizing, at the outset, the standardness with which the program must be followed is an important factor in getting a person through it smoothly.

Medical Approval Required

Before the participant is started on any part of the Purification program, he must first be given a medical exam and have written medical approval to do the program from an informed medical doctor.

Such an examination would include a check of the person's blood pressure, and a check for any symptoms of a weak heart or anemia.

The medical doctor also checks for any vitamin or mineral deficiencies the person may have and advises whatever vitamin and mineral supplements he should be taking to correct this, in addition to the vitamin/mineral regimen called for in the program.

Persons with physical conditions which might preclude their doing the standard Purification program (i.e., anyone who has a weak heart or anemia or even certain kidney conditions) may be given a similar program to be done on a much lower gradient.

Pregnancy and Breast Feeding

Pregnant women should not be put onto the Purification program. During pregnancy there is a certain amount of fluid exchange between the mother and the fetus, via the placenta.[3] Toxins which might have been lying dormant could, on the program, be released.

Some of these toxins, instead of being eliminated, could be

---

3. **placenta:** an organ that develops in the womb during pregnancy and supplies the fetus with nourishment.

transmitted to the fetus in a flow of fluids from the mother to the unborn child. There is no reason to risk the possibility of subjecting the unborn child to the effects of such toxins which, even if present but remaining dormant, might not otherwise reach him.

Similarly, mothers who are breast-feeding their babies should not do the program until the baby is no longer being breast-fed, as toxins released could be imparted to the baby in the mother's milk.

The Purification program would be done by the mother after the birth of the child and after any final medical check which pronounced the mother in good health and capable of undertaking the program. In the case of breast-feeding, the program would only be done when the baby had been completely weaned and was on his own formula.

Testing

A battery of tests can be done on the individual before and after the Purification program. These would include a personality test, IQ test, any available learning rate tests and others which would give a before-and-after picture of the person. Such before-and-after tests (quite in addition to any statements from the person himself) will often show up dramatic changes the person has made while on the program.

Other data taken before the participant begins the program would include, of course, a history of drugs, medicines or alcohol the person has had, his weight, blood pressure, any specific physical complaints or mental anxieties, and general details as to the state of the person's overall health.

The Program Case Supervisor *must* monitor the program

carefully on a daily basis, and this is done based on what the participant himself reports as well as by actual observation of the participant, as needed.

While on the program, the person is issued his vitamins, including niacin, minerals and oil, on a daily basis, and at the end of his running and sauna time each day he himself turns in a full written report of his progress. This is done on a daily report form provided him, which contains a checklist of items to be reported on. The daily report form would call for, at the very least, the following data:

1. How long he exercised.

2. How long he sweated in the sauna.

3. What vitamins were taken and in what amounts.

4. How much niacin was taken (in milligrams).

5. What minerals were taken and in what amounts.

6. How many glasses of Cal-Mag were taken.

7. Whether salt, potassium or bioplasma were taken and in what amounts.

8. How many glasses of water or other liquid (other than Cal-Mag) were taken.

9. Weight that day. (Include a note as to any weight gain or loss.)

10. Any somatics, restimulations, sensations, emotions, physical changes or other changes or occurrences experienced.

11. Any wins the person had on the program that day.

An individual folder must be kept for each program participant. The daily report is handed in to the Program Administrator who goes over it with the program participant to ensure that all points of the program were adhered to. The Administrator then places the report in the participant's folder and sends the folder to the Program Case Supervisor.

Daily Tight Supervision

The Program Case Supervisor must verify each person's daily progress and initial the person's report and any medical reports after he has inspected them. He then writes orders to correct any misapplication of any point of the program, such as skipping vitamins, not getting enough sleep, etc., as well as noting any increase in vitamin/mineral dosages that is to be made.

The folder is returned to the Program Administrator who personally takes up with the participant any changes to be made, such as increasing the niacin or other vitamin or mineral dosages. The Administrator also carries out any orders for correcting the participant, such as getting him back onto the proper schedule if he has gone off this, ensuring any errors are handled, and handles any questions the participant may have at any particular stage of the program.

Correct administration would include ensuring the participant never exercises or goes into the sauna alone, but carries out these actions with a partner.

Tight supervision would also include having blood pressure or other checks redone at intervals during the program, as needed.

2

Withdrawal from Drugs

2

Withdrawal from Drugs

The Purification program is not administered to those actively on drugs, though such persons need this program even more urgently, perhaps, than others. Thus, a workable withdrawal program must precede the Purification program for these individuals.

Such a program must be drugless and would include a substantial nutritional regimen.

Additionally, light counseling techniques (Objective Processes[1]), developed in the 1950s to extrovert a person's attention away from his body, have been put to effective use in helping people to get through withdrawal from drugs with a minimum of pain.

Also, quite in addition to the use of Cal-Mag in the healing and exchange processes involved in the Purification program,

---

1. **Objective Processes:** counseling procedures which help a person to look or place his attention outward from himself. *Objective* refers to outward things, not the thoughts or feelings of the individual. Objective Processes deal with the real and observable. They call for the person to spot or find something exterior to himself in order to carry out the procedures. Objective Processes locate the person in his environment, establish direct communication, and bring a person to present time, a very important factor in mental and spiritual sanity and ability.

calcium and magnesium provide a means of helping to handle withdrawal symptoms for persons coming off drugs.

Withdrawal Symptoms

The most wretched part of coming off hard drugs is the reaction called withdrawal symptoms. These are the physical and mental reactions to no longer taking drugs. They are ghastly. No torturer ever set up anything worse. People go into convulsions. These can be so severe that the addict becomes very afraid of them and so remains on drugs. The reaction can also produce death.

Until withdrawal procedures were developed, a drug patient had this problem:

    a. Stay on drugs and be trapped and suffering from there on out.

    b. Try to come off drugs and be so agonizingly ill meanwhile that he couldn't stand it.

It was a dead if you do, dead if you don't sort of problem.

Medicine did not solve it adequately. Psychotherapy certainly did not.

Handling Withdrawal

Fortunately, at least three approaches now exist for this problem:

    1. Light Objective Processes can ease the gradual withdrawal and make it possible.

2. Nutritional therapy, as sufficient vitamins and minerals assist the withdrawal.

3. Calcium and magnesium, taken in the Cal-Mag Formula.

So terrible can be withdrawal symptoms and so lacking in success have the medical and psychiatric fields been in dealing with them, that the full data on the use of the Cal-Mag Formula to counteract withdrawal symptoms should be broadly known.

The use of Cal-Mag, experimental in the early 1970s to help ease withdrawal symptoms, is now long past the experimental stage. Cal-Mag has been used very effectively during withdrawal to help ease and counteract the convulsions, muscular spasms and severe nervous reactions experienced by an addict when coming off drugs. The success of its application for withdrawal cases by drug rehabilitation centers such as Narconon has now been well established. Cal-Mag has been reported as effective in withdrawal from any drug, its effectiveness most dramatically observable with methadone[2] and heroin cases.

Methadone attacks bone marrow[3] and bones so one usually encounters a severe depletion of calcium in methadone users, characterized by severe pain in joints and bones, teeth problems, hair problems. Getting calcium into the system (in the acidic solution in which it can operate), along with magnesium for its effect on the nerves, helps to relieve these conditions.

---

2. **methadone:** a synthetic narcotic, similar to morphine but effective orally, used in the relief of pain and as a heroin substitute in the treatment of heroin addiction. Methadone failed as a "solution" to heroin addiction because people instead became addicted to methadone.

3. **marrow:** a soft fatty tissue in the interior cavities of bones that is a major site of blood cell production.

It has been reported that with use of Cal-Mag, a person can be withdrawn from methadone anywhere from two weeks to three months faster than without its use. This may apply in withdrawal from other drugs as well.

Since drugs or alcohol burn up the vitamin B_1 in the system rapidly, taking a lot of B_1 daily when coming off drugs helps to avoid the convulsions which often attend this deficiency. The B_1 must, of course, be flanked with other vitamin dosages to maintain a proper balance of needed nutrients. And, accordingly, sufficient quantities of Cal-Mag are needed, both to prevent created mineral deficiencies and to work its wonders in easing and relieving the agonies accompanying withdrawal.

From 1 to 3 glasses of Cal-Mag a day, with or after meals, *replaces any tranquilizer.* It does not produce the drugged effects of tranquilizers (which are quite deadly).

As calcium and magnesium are minerals, not drugs, one is not adding to the drug effects the person is already suffering from. Rather, one is providing those minerals which are certain to be in deficiency in such cases—and helping to provide some relief from the agonizing effects of such deficiencies.

3

More on Nutrition and Individual Schedule

3

More on Nutrition and Individual Schedule

$\mathbf{T}$ he following chapter contains data offered from a broad survey and review of cases in areas where the Purification program has been successfully delivered since its release.

Importance of Nutrition

What showed up throughout the survey data was the importance of the daily nutritional vitamins, minerals, oil, Cal-Mag and vegetables, and the role that these nutritional elements play in handling the traumatic[1] effects of restimulation of drugs and other toxins.

In each area it was observed that dropping out any of these supplements while on the program, skimping on them or taking them only sporadically, contrary to the program regulations, could create or intensify deficiencies which would then throw a curve into the program that would show up in any number of ways—tiring quickly, lack of energy, upset stomach, nausea, a general "not feeling good" or actually getting sick in some way, to name a few.

---

1. **traumatic:** distressing; emotionally disturbing.

Any omission of these standard elements was found to interfere with the progress and purpose of the program.

Many, many cases are now reported to have successfully completed the program under close supervision on the nutritional vitamin and mineral increases within the ranges given in the original research data.

Many areas report it has also been helpful to have a good familiarity with the books on nutrition written by the late Adelle Davis mentioned earlier in this text: *Let's Eat Right to Keep Fit, Let's Get Well, Let's Cook It Right* and *Let's Have Healthy Children* (all originally published by Harcourt, Brace Jovanovich, Inc., 737 Third Avenue, New York, NY 10017). These are among the most useful and popular compilations on the subjects of diet and biochemistry which have been published to date.

Don't Ignore Individual Tolerances

Where individual tolerances were taken into consideration and any vitamin imbalance or deficiency handled as stipulated in the regulations set forth in the program, the ranges published from the original research were reported to be highly workable for most.

In areas where the program has been successfully delivered, the person's originations[2] regarding his tolerance for or reactions to certain vitamins were never ignored. These would always be looked into and a correct solution worked out in alignment with the theory and factors of the program as originally researched.

---

2. **originations:** a coined word meaning statements or remarks volunteered by a person concerning himself, his ideas, reactions or difficulties; communications originated by the person himself.

In reported cases where the person was having some difficulty and some nutrient imbalance was the actual cause of the upset, where the vitamins and minerals were properly adjusted as above there was invariably improvement.

But it was necessary to *first* determine that the person actually was *taking* the vitamins and other nutritional elements he was supposedly taking and in what amounts, or if he was taking them only sporadically.

Responsibility of the Participant

It is the responsibility of the person who has undertaken to do the program to keep those overseeing the program well informed as to his daily actions and the results.

From all the reported data, it is not unusual at certain points of the program for some to protest a bit at the large quantities of vitamins to be taken. The protest is not in regard to results or benefits but simply in regard to the quantities to get down. While the niacin was always taken all at one time, in several areas it was found most viable to take the remainder of the vitamins at various intervals during the day, after meals or with snacks. One medical doctor has suggested that absorption of the needed nutrients is better accomplished in this way. The exception to this would be where one or more of the vitamins or minerals had been specifically suggested by the physician to be taken at certain set intervals.

Hidden "Diet" Factor

Also reported was the datum that there is a hidden factor to look for if a person is having difficulty and that is the person is not eating but is going along mainly on something like vitamins and niacin and yogurt alone. Or he has made some other major change in his eating habits. This was found in one area and totally explained why the person was having trouble on the program. It was then remedied by getting the individual onto regular and balanced meals.

Verbal Exchange Can Throw the Program Off

Departures such as those above were found quite often to come about as the result of exchange of verbal data or advice between participants on the program. This line must be watched to ensure the procedure is being followed as given, not someone else's version of it or some experimentation with it on his own.

Questions and Answers on Individual Scheduling

Can the program be completed satisfactorily on less than five hours daily? Where circumstances honestly prevented some persons from doing the program for five hours daily, a shorter time period was piloted.

It was found that the program could be completed effectively by some cases on less than five hours per day, provided the person *is getting benefit and change* on the shorter schedule.

The shorter schedules ranged from four hours down to a minimum of two and a half hours total running and sauna time daily. This period would then be spent as follows: twenty to thirty minutes of running and the remaining two hours or so in the sauna.

The same gradients applied when the person was on or starting a two-and-a-half-hour daily schedule as on any other schedule.

The approval of the Program Case Supervisor would be obtained for one to do the program on this shorter schedule, as there are other factors which enter into it. Any medical advice or order for the person to be on the shorter schedule would need to be followed.

The program can, and in most cases has, taken longer to complete on a shortened daily schedule, but survey results show that it can be done successfully by a good many people at a minimum of two and a half hours daily *provided all other points of the program are standardly maintained.*

Is the extent of a person's drug history a factor in the time spent daily on the Purification program? Per all the research and survey data assembled thus far, which is quite considerable, the extent of drug history is definitely a factor in determining how much time daily an individual would spend on the program.

Surveys show beyond any doubt that those with heavy or even mediumly heavy drug histories benefited most from the five-hour daily schedule. This can apply to persons with heavy medical drug histories as well as to those who have had heavy street drugs.

There are reports on record of persons with heavy drug histories who, though they had done fairly well at the beginning of the program on two and a half hours a day (with some phenomena turning on and dissipating[3]) did not begin to turn on restimulation of actual "trips" and blow through them until they were put onto a five-hour daily schedule.

Others reported that if something turned on while in the sauna they made it a point to stick carefully to the sauna time

---

3. **dissipating:** becoming scattered or dispersed; being dispelled; disintegrating.

(taking short breaks as necessary for water, salt or potassium or to cool off) until the manifestation vanished, and they then came out feeling good and refreshed. These same persons reported that if they short-cut the sauna time because something uncomfortable had turned on they came out feeling bad or dull and it would then take longer to go through the manifestation.

People with very light drug histories, as well, reported feeling calmer and more alert and cheerful after a stint in the sauna which was long enough to permit them to get through any restimulation or discomfort that had turned on.

There is everything to be said for putting a person on a schedule which will permit him to handle these factors, and it was found particularly important that those with heavy or mediumly heavy drug histories were scheduled properly so that they were able to get full return from the action and wind up with the expected end phenomena.

Who determines the schedule? On any questions as to daily schedule, the Program Case Supervisor would adjudicate as to the daily time period for the individual.

In any case where the person is on a special medical program, the physician's orders regarding schedule must be adhered to.

The first consideration regarding schedule would be what is going to give the person the most gain. Wherever possible the person would do the program for five hours daily and most people going through the program have done so on that schedule.

In instances where a shorter daily schedule was actually required for best results on some individuals, the schedule was adjusted accordingly.

In cases where persons honestly had limited time, these were considered for the minimum two and a half hour daily time period, as it would be more important for them to do the program than deny it to them. But it was necessary to ensure that each person could and did make progress on the shorter daily schedule as he continued it and, if not, to get him onto the regimen that was proper for him.

Some who started at two and a half hours daily later requested to move up to the five-hour period. There have also been cases where persons on the shorter schedule were getting heavy restimulation of drugs which they could not handle on the shorter period and, when switched to the five-hour period, they did remarkably better. This can occur, apparently, with street drug or medical drug users and is something to be borne in mind. Whenever possible the heavier drug cases were put on the five-hour schedule to begin with.

Again, correct gradient was the watchword[4] here, as in all other aspects of the program.

The supervising of cases on the program would not be done rotely but would always be done on an individual basis with the individual never pushed farther or faster than he could go. To do otherwise would be a violation of the technology of the program and a violation of the required gradients.

The successful action has been to get the person on a schedule where he is winning and getting change and able to handle what comes up, and then ensure he gets in that amount of time each day and *preferably at the same time each day.* Regularity of schedule plays a big part in completing the program smoothly and effectively.

---

4. **watchword:** a word or phrase expressive of a principle or rule of action; slogan.

Departures from Schedule Regularity

One of the factors examined closely in the course of this survey was whether or not there was a common sauna time limit for most people (within the recommended five hours) after which the person got tired and got less return for the remainder of the period.

By "less return" is meant simply nothing happening, but the person enduring the period on a "now I am supposed to" basis even though tired and feeling he had done all he could for one day.

In those cases where the program was being carried out very standardly, there were no reports of such tiredness setting in before the five hours were up (i.e., tiredness which was due to length of time spent in the sauna). Several cases reported they experienced tiredness as part of a restimulation of drug reactions, etc., but they were able to spot it as such and blow through it within the five-hour period.

However, there were a number of reports from individuals stating they did get tired in the sauna well within the five hours and got limited or no benefit from it beyond that tiring point. The daily time limits for gain reported by these cases varied widely from person to person, the reported limits ranging from four hours down to two and a half hours or less. The individual's drug history did not seem to be a factor, as the reports came from persons whose drug histories ranged from heavy down to few or no drugs, medical or otherwise.

These cases were looked into carefully and when all the pertinent data was examined, what showed up were departures from the standard procedure of the program.

The departures found were (in order of frequency):

a. Not enough sleep.

b. Insufficient salt or potassium or bioplasma taken while in the sauna or before running, *or* a combination of (a) and (b).

c. Dropped out vitamins that day, skimping on vitamins or minerals taking these sporadically.

d. An undetected and/or unhandled vitamin or mineral deficiency.

Correction of these factors brought about smoother progress and much improved results for these individuals.

Reactions

At best, any one of the above-listed factors or omissions could result in the person tiring too quickly, experiencing unnecessary discomfort, getting limited gain per hour and prolonging the program unnecessarily. The apparency would be that the program was not working when in actual fact it was not being applied standardly.

Where a person on *any* schedule reports he is tiring at a certain point and getting little or no benefit per hour spent beyond that point, one would need to determine if an adjustment of the daily time period was needed. But, as has been found, *additionally and always* one would carefully examine exactly what the person was doing on any section of the program and get any departures rectified.

Regardless of whether the person is on the maximum or

minimum daily schedule, departures from other aspects of the procedure would decrease the benefits until these departures were handled.

Program Interruption

Probably the biggest single factor found in keeping the person progressing smoothly on through to successful completion of the program was regularity of the actions. This includes regularity of the exercise and sauna schedule, nutrition and sleep.

Where any one part of the procedure was being done erratically it would throw the other parts out, or give that apparency, and the effect could sometimes be quite puzzling to the Program Case Supervisor or the medical doctor and others assisting in the administration of the program.

Per firsthand observation and data collected by report and survey, where people who had otherwise been doing well began skipping a day here or there, skimping or cutting down on the daily program time or missing sleep, it usually resulted in upset of some degree. They began to report "feeling bad" or feeling "sickish" or actually getting sick following some irregularity or disruption of the routine. Where this occurred, the discomfort or upset was more severe among those with heavier drug histories.

A possible explanation of this is that the process has been interrupted and one is getting a backlogging of the drug and other toxic effects rather than a routine release of these at the same rate as when the person was on schedule. Therefore, the person could be subject to a piling up of the restimulative effects of these at a rate not easily handled by him, and this could be further compounded by any continuation of an erratic schedule.

The handling was to get the person onto or back onto a proper and predictable daily regimen and maintain it through to completion of the program.

What was stressed here was that in this, as well as all parts of the Purification program, it is a matter of the person following the normal and generally accepted rules for good health. He would then be in the best possible shape to attain the benefits which are available to him.

4

Questions and Answers Regarding Program Completion

4

Questions and Answers Regarding Program Completion

In the course of the broad survey done several months after the Purification program was first released, certain questions and situations arose as to valid completion of the program. These are included here so that the data may be broadly known.

Niacin Reaction at Completion

One of the most common questions posed was:

Can the program be considered complete if the person seems to have reached the end phenomena and is getting no more reaction or manifestation turning on or no other change occurring but still gets a slight result from 5000 mg. niacin?

In such a case, the person could be hung up in some error in the early stages of the program, which would show up in a full review of his Purification program history. One could do a full inspection of his folder, particularly in the area of minerals and vitamins, what effect they had, whether the dosages were standard and kept in the proper balance, whether the program had been administered and followed standardly and regularly.

The participant should be interviewed as well, and one might find departures from the regimen, such as that he "doesn't like vegetables and never eats them," he has difficulty taking the oil so he skips it, or other similar omissions.

In other words, parts of the program could have been violated and this could be showing up in the manifestation described above. If the program hasn't been done standardly throughout, one could get such a situation.

It may be that he has a deficiency which has been over-looked and not handled and thus some sort of hang-up has been created. The point here is that there could be an unhandled deficiency which won't allow a complete discharge of the toxic residues.

If the folder shows irregularities a medical check would be done to determine if a deficiency exists and, if so, to get it remedied. Getting this handled and ensuring the program is continued with all of its regulations standardly in should then bring it to successful completion.

One must not overlook the possibility, however, that the person may simply have more to do on the program.

"Overrun"[1]

There is another possibility, and this may be the most common, which is that the person has reached the end phenomena, has continued past it, and is now "overrunning" the action. If he has done the program standardly and did, earlier,

---

1. **overrun:** the condition of continuing an action or a series of actions past the optimum point, or past the point where that action has ceased to produce change.

exhibit signs of valid completion which went unnoticed and unacknowledged, the chances are that he is complete on the program despite the fact he is still getting some slight result from 5000 mg. of niacin.

It is possible to overrun the program if one is not well aware of what is to be looked for in the end phenomena. There have been cases of overrun where the person was continued for some weeks at 5000 mg. (5 grams) of niacin with nothing more turning on than a very slight niacin flush effect. And there have been similar cases of overrun that occurred at less than 5000 mg. of niacin.

The possibility exists here that if the point of completion of the program (all drug and toxic residuals fully sweated out) is reached and bypassed the person could begin to dramatize[2] a niacin flush. The condition tends to hang up because it is not acknowledged or signalized to have ended. That is simply an educated guess as to one possible cause of the situation. But it is also borne out by careful study of several cases on record where bypass of the end phenomena and overrun did occur.

After the person has been on the regimen for some time, has come through good changes and is exhibiting all the indicators of being complete, carrying him on the program for six or seven days with no further effects at any dosage is really an overrun. In some of these cases it appears that 5000 mg. niacin isn't doing anything that 3500 mg. of niacin didn't do.

---

2. **dramatize:** repeat in action what has happened to one in experience; replay now something that happened then. *Dramatization* is the duplication of the content of a mental image picture, entire or in part, by a person in his present time environment. The degree of dramatization is in direct ratio to the degree of restimulation of the mental image pictures causing it. When dramatizing, the individual is like an actor playing his dictated part and going through a whole series of irrational actions. *See also* **mental image picture** and **restimulation** in the glossary.

To repeat, completion of the program can and has been reached on dosages of 5000 mg. niacin and on dosages of lower than 5000 mg. of niacin. Once the drug and chemical residuals are handled, they're handled. The person will feel the difference. Upping the dosage does not necessarily find more to be handled. And continuing the person past the valid completion can hang the whole thing up and produce a slight effect as a dramatization, either sporadically or each time the niacin is taken.

This can then become confusing to the person himself and those supervising the program. If the overrun is continued, you will see the person become less alert or dispirited,[3] even if slightly. His general appearance and demeanor[4] will be a bit less bright; he may become disheartened. He may now be attempting to produce some effect that isn't there to be had and begin to feel the action is interminable. Certainly the person will feel less enthusiastic about the whole procedure and may begin to protest it. The picture now looks as if the program is incomplete, whereas what has happened is that he achieved the end phenomena, reached a point where he felt great, was getting no further manifestations of any kind (if even only for a day) and the fact was not acknowledged but bypassed. Overrun phenomena then sets in. The handling is to acknowledge the person's completion of the program and end it off.

Overrun can also occur in quite a different way. One Program Case Supervisor reported he had had cases where the person, from all indications, was complete and stated that he was complete but wanted to continue a bit longer "just to make sure." Allowed to go on, these cases promptly got into overrun phenomena. They were getting no more change and became

---

3. **dispirited:** discouraged; dejected; disheartened; gloomy.

4. **demeanor:** conduct; behavior.

somewhat dispirited. In each of these cases, the end phenomena had actually been reached at the point the person stated he was complete.

Thus, it appears that on the Purification program it doesn't do to continue past the point of genuine completion. Should it happen, it is handled simply by having the person spot when he *did* complete, then fully acknowledging that and ending off on the program.

Another question that has come up with some frequency is:

What would account for a person who has genuinely completed the program with no niacin reaction at 5000 mg. (or less) then a short time later getting a reaction at lower niacin dosages?

Such a later reaction, where the person *has* actually standardly completed the program to its correct end phenomena, does not mean that the program is incomplete.

To understand this reaction, one needs a good understanding of mental image pictures and how they work. The specifics of what has happened in these instances can be quite variable, but what you are looking at here in general is that there has been an environmental shift or change which produced another type of mental image picture restimulation.

To begin with, we are living in a two-pole, two-terminal universe. It takes two terminals, positive and negative, to manufacture electricity. Magnets are also an example of the two-pole aspect of this universe: Every magnet has a north pole and a south pole which attract each other and create a magnetic field. This phenomenon can be observed in the operation of the mind as well—a person's mental image pictures on their own do not react on him continually; this only occurs when a mental image picture has been restimulated by some factor in the present environment which approximates part of that mental image picture.

It takes a two-terminal situation to hang something up. On the Purification program we are looking at a dual situation: one, the actual drugs and toxic residuals in the body and two, the individual's mental image pictures of the drugs and biochemical substances and their residues and his experiences from their effects.

As discussed in an earlier chapter of this book, the two conditions hang up in perfect balance, playing against each other.

On the Purification program, we break up this balance by flushing the actual toxic deposits out of the body. With the toxic deposits gone, the hang-up between the two conditions no longer exists. This then permits the constant restimulation of the mental image pictures to cease.

But what if the person experiences a niacin reaction shortly after he has validly completed the program? What could cause such a phenomenon?

The Purification program is designed to handle the actual toxic residues which may be lodged in the tissues, which by their presence and restimulative effects could hinder or slow a person's mental and spiritual advancement.

The Purification program is *not* meant to handle the individual's mental image pictures related to drugs and toxic substances. After the program is complete, these may not necessarily be in restimulation due to the presence of toxic residuals—but they are still there and may yet be restimulated by *other* factors.

As one example of this, a person who has finished the program but who is still taking niacin daily might restimulate mental pictures of a past sunburn by spending time out in the sun. With these mental pictures active once again, he may experience a flush when he takes his daily dose of niacin.

This doesn't automatically mean that the program was not really completed. It most often simply means that a mental picture or pictures have become active—nothing to be alarmed at, as they will in most cases simply become inactive again after a short while; from three to ten days is the most commonly observed interval. These mental pictures can be dealt with effectively through Scientology counseling, but such handling is beyond the scope of the Purification program and this book.

"Rabbiting"

Supervisors report there have been a few cases who "rabbited" (wanted to run away from continuing the program to completion because it was uncomfortable, or out of other considerations). These persons insisted they were complete after a very few days at low niacin dosage when little or nothing had yet turned on. But these cases were few and were easily detected and handled by bringing them to a better understanding of the program and its purpose. In two such cases where the person was mistakenly allowed to attest to completion after too brief and skimpy a run, both went into drug restimulation which should and would have been handled routinely on the program. After full review of these cases, with medical participation, they were put back on the program and completed it properly.

Judging from reports, including the many personal reports received, by far the majority of participants are eager to experience and handle and release those conditions which can show up on the Purification program. They report drugs, medicines, anesthetics, alcohol, restimulation of various other biochemical reactions, and somatics or other manifestations turning on, discharging and vanishing, and they report them all enthusiastically and with great relief—and look for more! Such cases will often know and tell you when they've honestly reached the end phenomena.

Trying to Handle "Everything"

What also showed up on the program was the rare bird[5] who would try or expect to handle on this program everything that had ever been wrong with him and who looked for some result above and beyond what the program is designed to accomplish. Such a case would need to be given a very thorough understanding of the program and its exact purpose, and his progress would be very carefully reviewed throughout. It is possible that with toxic residuals released from the body, other bodily conditions the person may be suffering from might then be treated with good success.

It was found important to make it real to any participant that all that is being looked for here is the person free from drug and toxic residuals and their restimulative effects, so as to make real mental and spiritual gains possible.

It is up to the Program Case Supervisor to know each case under his care, to be familiar with the progress of each case, to keep medical liaison lines in, and to know well the indicators

---

5. **bird:** a person, especially one having some peculiarity.

to expect when the person has achieved the end phenomena so that it can be acknowledged and validated.

Other Handling Tips

In successful application of the program, any bad indicators, odd or strange indicators or upset would be always picked up and handled at once.

If the person was in some heavy restimulation in the sauna and just wanted to get through it without interruption, he was not forced or badgered but permitted to go through it easily and gradually at his own rate and he would then come out the other side all right. Per reports, most people know when they are in a drug restimulation and will tell you.

In a case where the cause of the upset wasn't immediately obvious, the Program Administrator would simply sit down with the person and talk it over to find out what was going on.

What worked well was to have the participant read over all points of the program, or to have the Administrator take up each of these points with him, and the person himself would then very often spot and point out where he went off the rails. And, in most cases, he would prove to be right. It was very often found to be a matter of something having been altered or added or dropped out and this would be resolved by getting him back on the correct regimen and doing the program by the book.

If it doesn't appear to resolve, no guesswork or experimentation is done. The person must be given a medical check and any needed adjustment of his regimen then put in.

Summary

In summary, it has been found that there are any number of ways in which one can depart from the correct procedure and the effects of one such departure can be similar to or appear to be similar to those of another. This can make some cases look complicated indeed—and unnecessarily so. So it has also been found that it is vital to indoctrinate the participant on the standard actions of the program at the outset and then do everything possible to preserve that standardness throughout.

5

Drugs: Their Effects and Manifestations

5

Drugs: Their Effects and Manifestations

Various manifestations turn up on the Purification program and these can vary widely from person to person.

Anything from an insect bite to a full-blown restimulation of an LSD trip may turn on and these simply run themselves through and vanish as the program is continued.

In order to fully understand these manifestations, it is first necessary to know what drugs really *do.*

Drugs Are Poisons

Drugs are essentially poisons. The degree they are taken determines the effect. A small amount acts as a stimulant. A greater amount acts as a sedative. A larger amount acts as a poison and can kill one dead. This is true of any drug. Each has a different amount at which it gives those results.

Some drugs have a direct and specific effect upon a person's mind. Marijuana, peyote,[1] morphine, heroin, etc., apparently

---

1. **peyote:** a hallucinogenic drug prepared from the dried, buttonlike tops of a type of Mexican cactus.

---

turn on the mental image pictures one is stuck in, and turn them on hard. LSD, originally designed for psychiatric use, can reportedly make schizophrenics[2] out of normal people.

Though drugs are considered valuable by addicts to the degree they produce some "desirable effect," a person on drugs is dangerous to others around because he has blank periods. He has unrealities and delusions that remove him from present time.[3]

Drugs and Regression

Drugs tend to regress a person. That is to say, they tend to throw him out of present time and into his past. They can actually stick the person in periods of his past experiences, often past experiences with drugs, alcohol or medicine.

Drugs—LSD, marijuana, alcohol and the remainder of the long list—produce a threat to the body like any other poison. The threat is to the *body*. The being reacts by pulling in a mental image picture. Threatened with loss of a body, he pulls in a picture to put *something* there.

What he puts there is some mental image picture from the past, sometimes a combination of fancy and fact. He can do

---

2. **schizophrenics:** (*psychiatry*) persons who have *schizophrenia*, a major mental disorder typically characterized by a separation of the thought processes and the emotions, a distortion of reality accompanied by delusions and hallucinations, a fragmentation of the personality, motor (involving muscular movement) disturbances, bizarre behavior, etc. The word *schizophrenia* comes from Greek, meaning *split mind*.

3. **present time:** the time which is now, rather than in the past. It is a term loosely applied to the environment existing in the present. A person said to be "out of present time" would be someone whose attention is fixed on past events to such an extent that he is not fully aware of or in communication with his actual present environment.

---

this in some cases so hard that it becomes more real (and safer, in his estimation) than his present time.

Thus, under threat he goes out of present time. (What has actually happened is that he has pulled some of his mental image pictures from the past up into present time so these are affecting him in present time. But however one wants to view this, the truth of the matter is that he is at least partially acting and thinking and feeling not out of *this* moment but out of some moment in the past in which he is now stuck.)

A person's time track[4] is ordinarily made up of the re-corded moment-to-moment events experienced as he moves along through time. But when the person on drugs has pulled in pictures from the past his time track for this period is not being made up only of present time events. Instead, what is being recorded is a composite of past events, imagination and present events.

Thus, right there before your eyes he, apparently in the same room as you are, doing the same things, is really only partially there and partially in some past event.

He *seems* to be there. But really he isn't tracking fully with present time.

What is going on, to a rational observer, is *not* what is going on to him. Thus he does not duplicate statements made by another but tries to fit them into his composite reality. In order to fit them in he has to alter them.

He may be *sure* he is helping you to *repair* the floor when in

---

4. **time track:** the consecutive record of mental image pictures which accumulates through a person's life. *See also* **mental image pictures** in the glossary.

actual fact what you are doing is cleaning the floor. So his actions (which seem logical and correct to him) are actually hindering the operation in progress. Thus, when he "helps you" mop the floor he introduces chaos into the activity. Since he is *repairing* the floor, a request to "give me the mop" gets reinterpreted as "hand me the hammer." But the mop handle is larger than a hammer, so the bucket gets upset, with suds and water splashed all over the place.

That is a mild example—the kind of thing that doesn't make the headlines. But what of the accidents, the crimes, the despair that leads to all manner of tragedies that do make the headlines?

As a being can come up with an infinity of combinations, there would be an infinity of types of reactions to drugs.

What is *constant,* however, is that he is *not running in the same series of events* as others.

This can be slight, wherein the person is seen to make occasional mistakes. It can be as serious as total insanity where the events apparent to him are *completely* different than those apparent to anyone else. And it can be all grades in between.

It isn't that he doesn't know what's going on. It is that he perceives *something else* going on instead of the actual present time series of events that is going on.

Painkillers

In 1969 I made a breakthrough on the action of painkillers (such as aspirin, tranquilizers, hypnotics[5] and soporifics[6]).

5. **hypnotics:** agents or drugs that produce sleep; sedatives.

6. **soporifics:** things that cause sleep, as medicines or drugs.

At that time it had never been known in chemistry or medicine (and I am not sure that it is generally known today) exactly how or why these things worked. Such compositions are derived by accidental discoveries that "such and so depresses pain."

The effects of existing compounds are not uniform in result and often have very bad side effects.

As the reason they worked was unknown, very little advance has been made in biochemistry. If the reason they worked were known and accepted, possibly chemists could develop some actual compounds which would have minimal side effects.

Pain or discomfort of a psychosomatic[7] nature comes from mental image pictures. These are unknowingly created by the person himself and they impinge[8] or impress against the body.

By actual clinical test, the actions of aspirin and other pain depressants are to:

A. *Inhibit the ability of the being to create mental image pictures,*

and also

B. *To impede the electrical conductivity of nerve channels.*

With this, the person is rendered stupid, blank, forgetful, delusive, irresponsible. He gets into a "wooden" sort of state,

---

7. **psychosomatic:** *psycho* refers to mind and *somatic* refers to body; the term *psychosomatic* means the mind making the body ill or illnesses which have been created physically within the body by derangement of the mind.

8. **impinge:** make an impression; have an effect or impact.

---

unfeeling, insensitive, unable and definitely not trustworthy, a menace to his fellows, actually.

When the drugs wear off or start to wear off, the ability to create starts to return and *turns on somatics much harder.* One of the answers a person has for this is *more* drugs. To say nothing of heroin, there are, you know, aspirin addicts. The compulsion stems from a desire to get rid of the somatics and unwanted sensations again. There is also some evidence of dramatization of the pictures turned on from earlier drug taking. The being gets more and more wooden, requiring more and more quantity and more frequent use of the drug.

To paraphrase an old adage,[9] we used to have iron men and wooden ships. We now have a drug society and wooden citizens.

If one were working on this biochemically, the least harmful pain depressant would be one that inhibited the creation of mental image pictures with minimal resulting "woodenness" or stupidity, and which was body-soluble so that it passed rapidly out of the nerves and system. There are no such biochemical preparations at this time.

The medical aspect is an understandable wish to handle pain. Doctors should press for better drugs to do this that do not have such lamentable[10] side effects. Drug companies would be advised to do better research. The formula of least harmfulness is that given above.

---

9. **adage:** a traditional saying expressing a common experience or observation; proverb.

10. **lamentable:** deplorable; regrettable.

Burn-up of Vitamin Reserves

Drugs can also temporarily stimulate (before they ruin them) body glands. And they can produce momentary feelings of well-being or what is known as "euphoria." Part of this is probably caused by the fact that they shut off, temporarily, the painful mental image pictures from the past.

They can also speed up the burning of reserves of vitamins. A drug or alcohol rapidly burns up the vitamin B_1 in the system. Certain drugs also burn up all available niacin and vitamin C. This speeded burn-up can also bring about a temporary feeling of well-being; it adds to the "happy state."

But when the system is out of B_1, the person becomes depressed. When the reserves are gone, the delusions called delirium tremens ("dt's") or the withdrawal symptoms that follow are nightmarish indeed.

"If You're Numb Nothing Can Hurt You"

Drug users, from observation, are apparently sitting on the fallacy that "if you're numb nothing can hurt you." Drugs, then, are probably a defense against the physical universe.[11]

They do block off pain and other unwanted sensations. But there is a whole sector of *desirable* sensations and drugs block off *all* sensations.

Sexually it is common for someone on drugs to be very stimulated at first. This is the "procreate[12] before death" impulse, as

---

11. **physical universe:** the material universe, which is made up of matter, energy, space and time.

12. **procreate:** beget or generate (offspring).

---

drugs are a poison. But after the original sexual "kicks,"[13] the stimulation of sexual sensation becomes harder and harder to achieve. The effort to achieve it becomes obsessive while it itself is less and less satisfying. In spite of propaganda[14] to the contrary, even sexual sensation is blocked off with drugs and this is true even after drugs have apparently heightened it for one or two times. After that it is dead, dead, dead.

Emotion, Perception and Somatic Shut-off

Those who have been long and habitually on drugs, medicine or alcohol sometimes suffer from emotional, perception or somatic shut-offs. They appear anesthetized (unfeeling) and sometimes have "nothing troubling them," whereas they are in reality in a suppressed physical condition and cannot cease to take drugs or drink or medicine.

Any such case took up drugs, medicine or alcohol because of unwanted pain, sensation or misemotion.[15] The person looked on drugs, alcohol or medicine as a cure for unwanted feelings.

The only brief[16] that can be held out for drugs is that they

---

13. **kicks:** thrills; pleasurable excitement.

14. **propaganda:** information, ideas or rumors deliberately widely spread to help or harm a person, group, movement, institution, nation, etc.

15. **misemotion:** a coined word that is used to mean an emotion or emotional reaction that is inappropriate to the present time situation. It is taken from *mis-* (wrong) + *emotion*. To say that a person was *misemotional* would indicate that the person did not display the emotion called for by the actual circumstances of the situation. Being misemotional would be synonymous with being irrational. One can fairly judge the rationality of any individual by the correctness of the emotion he displays in a given set of circumstances. To be joyful and happy when circumstances call for joy and happiness would be rational. To display grief without sufficient present time cause would be irrational.

16. **brief (hold a brief for):** support or defend by argument; endorse.

give a short, quick oblivion from immediate agony and permit the handling of a person to effect repair. But even this is applicable only to persons who have no other system to handle their pain.

Dexterity,[17] ability and alertness are the main things that prevent getting into painful situations and these all vanish with drugs.

So drugs set you up to get into situations which are truly disastrous and keep you that way.

Drugs versus Learning

Drugs impede learning. In view of all the other things drugs do, one might easily deduce this. But the statement is more than simply a deduction, it is empirical[18] fact. Learning rate—the length of time it takes someone to learn something—has been proven to be slower in drug users than others. Actual tests show that the learning rate of a person who has been on drugs is much lower than that of a person who hasn't.

Drugs, then, would prevent a person from becoming educated. Now let's weigh this against the fact that drug usage among students is not only tolerated in many schools and colleges, but some drugs are even *employed* in certain schools—one example being psychiatrists advocating and pushing the use of dangerous, addictive drugs as a means to handle what are termed "hyperactive" children.

This may, indeed, be the root of the foul-up of current

---

17. **dexterity:** skill or adroitness in using the hands or body; agility; also, mental adroitness or skill; cleverness.

18. **empirical:** derived from or guided by experience or experiment.

education which has been so widely publicized in recent years. Teachers have been cited, in various articles in the press and other media, for failure or inability to teach. But the problem, at its root, may not be the teachers at all.

Whatever the actual statistics may be on that score, certain it is that drugs are prevalent in schools. And certain it is that drugs impede learning and thus impede education.

And a civilization that cannot be educated, that cannot learn, cannot last. This means *this* civilization will be ended unless we do something about it.

Learning Rate and Criminality

Where drugs are impeding learning, discipline would also be nonfunctional.

The memory of a person who is on or has been on drugs is often such as to remove him from fear of consequences for any of his actions. The answer, one might think, is discipline. But discipline is enforced learning. If attempts to simply teach the value of ethics fail in the face of impeded learning, attempts to teach by discipline and justice actions—enforced learning—fail even harder. The person who can't learn and who is then subjected to attempts to force learning by disciplinary action simply becomes criminal.

What good does it do a government to try to get police and justice actions into effect in a society that cannot learn? Governmental threats, in a society that cannot learn, would be of no use. The society would not learn from them; therefore it wouldn't matter what measures the government took. A society that could not learn that was then subjected to attempted enforced learning would, in the end, become criminal.

Manifestations

As a person sweats out the residual drugs in his system on the Purification program, any number of manifestations can occur. Such manifestations can be the result of one's use of or exposure to *any* chemical substance or drug which has then lodged, in whatever minute residual amount, in the cells or tissues of the body.

Incoming reports and medical case histories abound in statements from participants on the program where the person identified the reactions he was getting with past on-the-job experiences or occurrences in his life in general.

They include, for example, reports of toxic exposure to vinyl paints, insecticides, paint thinner, a wide variety of industrial chemicals, preservatives, plant sprays and the like. Some have turned on sensations which they recognize or identify with previous dental experiences, X-ray treatment, dental anesthetics such as novocaine or anesthetics for various operations, or any of the sensations accompanying various physical ills or injuries for which some type of medicine or drug was used.

This includes, of course, in no small measure, experiences with street drugs or what are now termed in some quarters "recreational" drugs, such as marijuana, cocaine, heroin, hashish,[19] LSD, etc. If there are drug residues to be flushed out it is not uncommon for the person to experience a restimulation of the exact effects from the drug or medicine when he first took it.

---

19. **hashish:** a drug made from the resin contained in the flowering tops of hemp, chewed or smoked for its intoxicating and euphoric effects.

Thus, one might expect to encounter manifestations related to medical or pharmaceutical chemicals, patent medicines,[20] industrial or household chemicals as well as from any experience he may have had with hard street drugs. And this apparently can extend to any nutritional deficiency, or illness as a result of such deficiency, which has been caused by the ingestion or absorption of any of these chemical substances.

Aches, Pains, Somatics

Old injuries or old somatics may turn on, flare up[21] for a brief spell and then vanish. These may be sharply defined and easily recognized by the individual as related to some former experience, or simply vague feelings of discomfort which are not identified as relating to any one specific illness or injury or accident. They might range from headaches, to muscular spasms, muscular aches, swellings, skin rashes, hives, bronchial[22] symptoms or any of a number of other aches, pains or somatics.

Sensations

Participants have reported the following sensations while sweating out residuals in the sauna: Light, "cloudy" feelings in the head, floating sensations, dizziness, feelings of being "spaced-out,"[23] numbness—often in the mouth and around gums or in some instances in the limbs or extremities,

---

20. **patent medicines:** medicines sold without a prescription in drugstores or by sales representatives, and usually protected by a trademark.

21. **flare up:** begin again suddenly, especially for a short time after a quiet time.

22. **bronchial:** of or pertaining to the bronchi, any of the major passageways of the lungs; especially either of the two main branches of the trachea, or windpipe.

23. **spaced-out:** dazed or stupefied because of the influence of narcotic drugs.

"hung-over"[24] feelings, or any of the feelings accompanying street drugs.

Periods of intoxication—drunkenness—have reactivated briefly for some individuals while in the sauna, and then dissipated and vanished. Persons who have experienced radiation while living in areas of atomic bomb testings or fallout,[25] and some who were in the armed services in Vietnam who were subject to the defoliant, Agent Orange, have done the Purification program with some very interesting results and tremendous relief reported.

Smells and Tastes

Very often the person will reexperience the smell or taste of some particular substance. Some of those described by program participants are: a metallic taste, an ether[26]-like smell, the taste of novocaine, "a bitter taste," a "medicine-like" taste, a "chemical-like" taste, a marijuana smell, to name just a few of those which have been reported.

These can show up, too, as unusual body odors emitted during periods of sweating in the sauna.

An example is one participant who had worked for some time as a lifeguard at a swimming pool containing chlorinated water. For a certain period on the program, while in the sauna, he exuded sweat with such a strong and overpowering smell of chlorine that others had to temporarily leave the sauna!

---

24. **hung-over:** of or pertaining to the disagreeable physical aftereffects of drunkenness, such as a headache or stomach disorder, usually felt several hours after cessation of drinking.

25. **fallout:** the descent to earth of radioactive particles, as after a nuclear explosion or reactor accident; also the radioactive particles themselves.

26. **ether:** a drug used to produce anesthesia, as before surgery.

Emotions

Emotions which have been shut off or suppressed may start to reappear. The person may go through emotional reactions connected with past biochemical experiences and these reactions will then dissipate. The individual may also go through a period of dullness or stupidity and, as he comes through it, become more aware. He may find he can then do actions more easily and consequences may start to take on a new meaning for him. Memory can return.

Differences and Changes in Intensity

From reports based on direct observation, apparently what can happen in some cases (not all) is that the residuals of several past drugs and other chemicals (sometimes every drug or medicine the person has taken) can restimulate simultaneously and turn on heavily in the first week or ten days of the program at lower dosages of, say, up to 1000 mg. of niacin.

Others will experience these effects in a more graduated sequence, one following the other.

It doesn't always happen in an orderly fashion and in some instances it can be more severe than in others. But as the person sweats out the drug residuals and goes through any accompanying manifestations, the effects tend to become lighter and eventually no effects will show up even on the higher amounts of niacin.

A given manifestation may turn on, may or may not intensify, and then vanish wholly or partly in any one day. Then it may turn on again the following day, but less intensely. If one increases the vitamin and mineral dosage at this time, the manifestation is likely to turn on again, but it will be milder. These things don't become more and more severe day by day; they become less and less so day by day, providing the Purification program is continued properly.

At length the vitamins, minerals and other program actions no longer turn the manifestation on at all; it is gone. There is evidence that no amount of vitamin and mineral dosage above a certain final level for that individual will turn the manifestation on again.

Correct Gradient Is the Key

The trick is to take a proper gradient with the vitamins and mineral dosages. When these are administered in too steep a gradient a manifestation can turn on awfully hard, so the correct gradient must be kept in. And one must not "chicken out"[27] and discontinue the program with manifestations still occurring, either.

From the original research and piloting of this program, from reports of those subsequently delivering it and from personal reports of those who have completed it, one can expect any variety of manifestations to come up, not all of them comfortable by any means. There seems to be no set limit as to the variety of effects which can appear as the toxic residuals are released.

However, where the person was on a sensible and well-kept schedule, with correct nutrient dosages and all other parts of the program followed, these manifestations would deintensify and disappear without hanging up and without undue[28] discomfort

---

27. **chicken out:** stop doing something because of fear; decide not to do something after all even though previously having decided to try it.

28. **undue:** unwarranted; excessive.

for the person. In other words, an individual will experience the effects caused by any nutritional deficiencies as well as the restimulative effects of the toxic substances as they become active and discharge, but he comes through these periods satisfactorily on a standard program.

As long as the precautions listed earlier are well taken and the procedure followed exactly as given, the solution to any manifestation that turns on is to continue the program as outlined, with the manifestation diminishing—becoming less frequent, less intense—until it ceases altogether.

Appendix

A. An Examination of Purification
   Program Results

B. Where to Do the Purification
   Program

Appendix A

An Examination of Purification Program Results

Compiled by the Editors

Since 1979, when L. Ron Hubbard fully developed the breakthrough he called the Purification program, two major factors—indeed trends—have been contributing to the phenomenal popularity of the program. The first is the growing public awareness of the alarming extent to which we are faced with chemical bombardment and long-term toxic and drug residue build-up in our bodies. The second factor is the program's *results.* From testimonials to scientifically controlled experiments, the benefits claimed by people from all parts of the world who have experienced the program are routinely spectacular and well worth reporting.

The editors have assembled a sampling of just some of thousands of reports from people who have completed the program.

There is no claim made regarding what the program will specifically do for any one person. However, such things as enormously increased energy, faster learning rate, new levels of mental concentration, freedom from dependence on chemicals, substantially better perception capabilities, a greater feeling of general well-being as well as improvements in a broad range of health categories, are the types of reports that are commonplace among the tens of thousands of people who have completed the Purification program.

I remember what I was like prior to taking drugs. I was full of life and energy and dreams. Life was very clear and uncomplicated. I had a very good family life—one in which I loved and trusted my parents. I also had close friends that I enjoyed real relationships with as I was growing up. More than anything I wanted to be happy and have a game to play in which I would win.

But something happened along the way. I got involved with drugs. I was not trying to destroy myself—drugs were the "in" thing—to many people in my generation they were considered part of the "answer." It was too late by the time I realized that drugs were destroying my life. I had become "spaced-out" from drugs, detached very much from life itself. Those things that I had held precious in my youth— family, morality and honest friendships—were a thing of the past. Really caring about life and other people were beyond my grasp. What relationships I did have became superficial.

I remember wondering if I could ever really care about someone again. I was scared, as I realized that I was not the same person I had been before drugs. I was not as sharp, my mind was a fog. I was bitter and untrusting. If there was one part of my life that I wanted to change it was the fact that I had done drugs. There was not a day that went by that I did not worry about this. This only heightened my despair as I knew that I couldn't turn back time. Even after quitting drugs entirely I remained aware of the fact that I was not the same person that I had been before. The guilt, bitterness and sorrow was staggering.

Then I did L. Ron Hubbard's Purification program. I have now handled the effects of the drugs that I had taken. I got my energy back and I am no longer walking around in a fog. I can think clearly and my mind is quick and decisive again. I have my drive back and I'm a part of life. I feel real emotions again that have been shut off for years. I can confront having real and honest relationships with others and I'm restoring those which I lost. In fact I feel as if I have to make up for lost time as I have wasted away years of my life. Now I want to be able to do something constructive with every minute.

I only hope that everyone else who has been involved with drugs, be they street drugs, medicinal drugs, etc., has the same opportunity as I have had and that they do this program. It will change their lives for the better, and there is an awful lot of good that can be done with one's life to have that ruined by drugs. L. Ron Hubbard's Purification program performed a miracle for me. It gave me back my life and I am living proof of that. B.D.

Ability to Think Clearly

I feel totally in present time and totally in control of my attention—no more wandering thoughts or broken attention spans. Mental computations are now crystal clear and lightning fast. J.D.

Yes! I have finished the Purification program. The greatest thing about it was I knew I was finished. The symptoms are unmistakable—thinking clearer, feeling light and energetic, even handled my insomnia problem to a considerable degree. Quality of sleep vastly improved! F.L.R.

I definitely feel the Purification program has been a great help to me physically, mentally and emotionally. I haven't felt this good in quite a while. I am able to think a lot clearer, sleep better and get along with my fellow man better. This has been a giant step in my recovery from drugs. R.G.

Increased Energy

I cannot believe it!!! My body is energetic, I am no longer dependent on coffee, sugar or any other stimulant (I had a terrible problem of physical ups and downs before the program and felt dependent on some type of stimulant). I am much more calm and relaxed, and my whole outlook on life has changed; it seems almost unbelievable. I am happier than I've ever been. This is the first time in seven years I feel like I can (and I want to) really create my future. I feel like a new person. Seven years ago was when I first had a large amount of "heavy" drugs (actually I never was a heavy drug user—the heaviest being only marijuana, codeine for tonsillitis and novocaine). But it was after that point that I was never quite the same. The marijuana had a bad effect on me and those things that turned on never left . . . until now. [Now] I am calm, relaxed, ready to create and expand a new life. A.S.

It's just amazing how you can go along day to day and think you are functioning optimumly when actually you are dull and not up to par at all—it is so subtle that you really don't realize what is affecting you until you do the Purification program and find out what it feels like to no longer be under the influence of anesthetics. If anyone had told me that I was going around half-unconscious all the time I wouldn't have believed them. But that's the state I was in. Actually from the first time I had an anesthetic as a child—ether when I had my tonsils removed and then each operation after that just built up the anesthetics in my system. Sometimes it was an effort to be active, and [since completing the Purification program] that is totally gone. What a program— when you think of how many people are out there walking around feeling sort of dull and listless and just thinking they are just getting old or this and that reason for it—it's really incredible. Prior to the Purification program I used to get periods of being very tired and always attributed it to working too hard, etc. With the anesthetics totally out of my system I have not had any occurrence of this "tired old" feeling. I am bright and feel that my thinking processes are at their optimum. L.H.

Before I started the Purification program I was tired most of the time. I needed a lot of sleep and my body was always tired and out of tune.[1] Now, after the Purification program, I always feel energetic. I get up earlier and I always am rested. My body just feels great and that has helped me a lot because I can work a lot and I don't get tired. C.D.

---

1. **out of tune:** not in proper harmony or accord; unresponsive.

Enthusiasm toward Life

I'm clean! It feels fantastic! Not only does my body feel great but I have increased my certainty and am able to see. It's amazing how alive I feel. C.D.

This has been a truly fantastic program. I had many and various diseases, maladies, aches and pains and symptoms turn on and disappear, and I am grateful to feel physically sound and able to take care of a body. But I think the most spectacular gains were not physical. I feel brighter, more enthusiastic about life. My memory has improved. I don't feel confused or jumbled up. I'm sure I will be able to study better, too. B.K.

I can think much more clearly. I have a better balance emotionally. I am more calm and peaceful. I have a more positive attitude toward life and feel I can handle anything. R.V.

Increased Perception of the Environment

Have you ever had the experience of driving a car with a dirty windshield? You keep straining to see, you stop and rub at it with a cloth, you just can't get it clean so you keep going, hoping you'll be able to see. What a relief to get the glass really clean, so you can really see out! The Purification program is just like that, for your body. It removed chemicals and drugs from more than twenty years back that have had their unpleasant, recurring effects on me all this time. One of the best and most surprising results of this program is that my nearsightedness has actually improved—*I have to get less powerful lenses for my eyes. It's like getting a new body.*

My vision has become brighter and improved. My taste is much sharper and some things even taste completely different now, through a purified body. I would recommend the Purification program HIGHLY to ANYONE. M.C.

I just completed the Purification program and I feel fantastic. My body moves easily instead of being sluggish. I no longer have those "pictures" which used to confuse me. Now they're gone and there's nothing between me and what I observe. I am happier and more self-confident. L.M.

Along with the many other changes and benefits I experienced from the Purification program is one very important thing. My eyesight is improved, especially my night vision. Before, I feel I was 80 percent blind at night. Now it may be only 15 percent. I'm not a doctor but I'm the guy who has to look out of these two eyes and it is improved. R.H.

After completing the program all my main senses seemed improved—hearing, smell, taste, touch. And I have more strength in my hands than I used to have. I am a lot more stable, and more myself than ever before. P.G.

Mental Acuteness

Since having finished the Purification program my ability to study has increased about double plus. My ability to spot and handle things I don't understand has gotten very acute. There is a lot less hesitancy to dive into some theory or do some practical drill that I have never done before or am not familiar with, due to the fact of seeing things more clearly and just seeming to have a quicker ability to compute and duplicate correctly what it actually is I am studying. L.W.

It is much easier to concentrate on the study materials. My ability to understand what I've read is much increased. I can picture what the author is saying, making it much easier to read. V.L.

Before doing the Purification program, I was a medium student. I would study and get something out of it, but sometimes it was hard to get a concept or to understand a subject easily and understand every aspect of that subject. With the program now done, I feel I'm better at studying. It's easy for me to understand anything. I grasp the meanings of things in an instant. I even feel more intelligent and I have become one of the best students on my courses. C.D.

Feeling Clean and Healthy

I recently completed the Purification program and I must say it was the best cleansing program I've ever been on. Before doing the program I had been on diets, done exercise programs and fasted in an effort to cleanse my body of the toxins and impurities. But on all these programs, the residual deposits of drugs in the body were never addressed and so I continued to be affected by them. For instance, I'd go running and jog loose some residual effects of sodium pentothal[2] from a previous tooth extraction and I'd feel faint for a few seconds at a time intermittently over the next few weeks. On the Purification program my circulation improved greatly and I sweated out all residual drug deposits. The proof of this to me is how I feel now. None of the previous "side-effects" of drugs occur anymore when I exercise and am heavily active! I feel really healthy! M.J.M.

There is no doubt in my mind that this Purification program has made considerable improvements in my body in spite of the abuses to it during the past 67 years! L.J.

Physically I feel much better since being on the Purification program. My appetite is under my control. Before, I would go on eating binges. Now I don't. I eat what I want but it's not too much and I eat more healthful foods. My skin, which broke out badly the first time I came off drugs, has cleared up a lot. It's now on the road to recovery. I feel much better about myself and my body. S.U.

At first when I started the Purification program I didn't think much would happen—and the first few days nothing much did happen. Then all of a sudden I got sick for no apparent reason one night and it felt really good to go into the sauna the next day and

---

2. **sodium pentothal:** a yellowish-white drug injected intravenously as a general anesthetic and hypnotic.

sweat it out, plus the change in vitamins gave my body more of a chance to handle getting sick. I could actually feel the toxic poisons and past drugs I had taken coming out of my body. The nauseousness, headaches, aches and pains, usually didn't last very long and as long as I didn't stop doing my normal routine they would come out and dissipate with no problems. The main thing is that every time I would feel just a little bit (or a lot) stronger, healthier, cleaner—it was like growing a new body. L.W.

Recovery from Drugs

I have just participated in a miracle. I would never have believed that I would ever feel this good again. The Purification program saved my life, my soul, and in addition has made me a better human being. T.K.

My Purification program is finally complete and without a doubt I'd call it a complete success. I originally did it because I wanted to kick the drug scene, as well as my inability to do good in school. What I've gotten out of it is much, much more. I can now face up to everyday life and its problems without having to depend on a "crutch" to get me through the day. I've known for a long time that for me to get ahead in this world, I had to get out and do it myself, because nobody is going to do it for me. That's where drugs hurt me. They kept me from being able to do it on my own. Now I've finally escaped from that prison and can go on living my life the way it should be. Until now I hadn't even looked past college. Now, I'm looking way ahead to what I have to do and my dreams and aspirations. I enjoy being "straight"[3] now, whereas before I hated it. N.S.

Having completed the Purification program I feel fantastic. I feel like a teenager. I know my body is clean. I feel lighter and it's great to move my body with no effort. I've realized that this is the way my body is supposed to feel and I don't want to put anything into it to make it dirty. My mind is also bright and clear. I now can remember things. D.M.

I could feel that the drugs are all out. I know for a fact that I wouldn't take drugs no more. M.I.

I've cleaned my body and my mind of drugs. I feel physically fine. My sleep is back and I want to get on the right track. N.N.

I feel as though I have more energy. My cravings to get loaded[4] are not as intense as they were a few months ago. Most of the time I am not even thinking about it. I am feeling emotions I have not felt in some time. When I first got started my feelings were numb. Now I can feel anger, love, etc. I can remember things now and I don't space thoughts out like I used to. Overall, I just feel good. J.R.

It was a real high to see the changes taking place in my mind and body on a day-to-day basis. My sleep has come back to normal which is a big win for me. It is also great to get off the confusion and disorientation you have with drugs. J.K.

---

3. **straight:** (*slang*) free from using narcotics.

4. **loaded:** (*slang*) under the influence of alcohol or drugs.

Popularity among Performing Artists and Athletes

Upon entering this program, I had a vague, disoriented state of mind from many years of social [drug] abuse due to the business I am in. Approximately one third through the program, I felt my mind quite obviously becoming clearer than it's been for several years. Halfway through, my color perception and audio perception improved. This lucid[5] state of mind enhanced my creative attitude. At the end of the program I was awakening continuously, every day with this wonderful state of being. S.P. Songwriter, Composer, Recording Artist

My relations with other people in work and in my personal life have been cleaner. My skin has been greatly improved. My body feels cleaner and more revitalized. My perspective on life seems to be more motivated and clear. Problems don't seem as upsetting. I can establish my priorities with more focus. Definitely feel more centered. L.S. Dancer

My whole life—emotional and physical—has improved with the starting and completing of this program. I'm able to deal confidently with unpredictable circumstances, as well as the routine situation that might have caused me trouble in the past. My mind's more alert, and my body feels better than it has in years. K.K. Musician

Improved disposition, an overall feeling of well-being, wonderfully smooth skin. I feel like a million dollars! S.A. Actress

---

5. **lucid:** characterized by clear perception or understanding; rational or sane.

Less hours sleep. Better sense of humor. Skin glow. Better focus. Better attitudes towards handling problems. F.A. Actor

The spacey[6] feeling I used to get when under stress has disappeared. Completely. I feel I can now think about the rest of my life; whereas before I was constantly thinking of my health. My skin feels better and I have been told that I look better than before. H.R. Musician

I am calm, clear, focused. I fall asleep quickly and wake up early. As an athlete I am much more focused and light. My reflexes are improved, as well as the ability to "trust" my body's trained instinctive responses. There seems to be more time within each moment, an easy anticipation that seems almost precognitive.[7] I feel much more centered in life . . . I feel a much stronger sense of self, which I'm confident will enhance my artistic and professional life. Before the program I was losing interest in everything. [Now] the artist has returned from exile. Thanks! R.S. Actor

The whites of my eyes are clear for the first time in years. My skin looks terrific. My respiratory problems have cleared up—feels much "clearer." I feel stronger mentally and physically. U.P. Actress

Body and mind are in greater harmony—no desire to return to polluted state. Physical shape has improved,

---

6. **spacey:** same as *spaced-out:* dazed or stupified.

7. **precognitive:** having knowledge of a future event or situation, especially through extrasensory means.

---

eyes feel "sharp," mind is quicker, more directed. I feel more mellow about external events; sense of humor has increased. A greater sense of "timing" in regards to stunt work; undercurrent of joy, smiling more often. Aware of stress and how it manipulates my body. I am making efforts to eliminate stress stimulations from my existence. Less time spent in "mindless habit" behavior. K.K. Stuntwoman

It's been more of an uplift knowing that my body is cleared of toxic materials. I felt very light and energetic after each session, but most of the benefits I feel will be seen from here on out in my daily activity and accomplishments. For me, the program was an inner experience, and now I'm ready to see how it relates to my outer self. M.Y. Professional tennis player

A regaining of memory. Better attitude. A healthy feeling. Cleaned out. Better judgment. F.M. World champion motorcyclist

Radiation: Case Histories

Reports have also been received which detail the results of the Purification program on people with a history of radiation exposure. One physician reported this when he completed the program:

Prior to starting the Purification program, I had a history of moderately heavy radiation exposure. This consisted of long periods of sun exposure through childhood and college and frequent X-ray exposure from working around X-ray machines with patients for some seven-odd years. I had no physical problems or complaints upon starting the Purification program. My drug history had been very light. During the program I had several episodes of extreme flush, splotchy rashes accompanied by nausea and a very solid, wooden feeling. At times, there was an electrical kind of discharge from the body especially to the arms and hands. Interesting enough, after the program I realized several low-grade somatics that I previously had ignored were gone. Small things, like occasionally unexplained nausea or mild aches in the muscles and joints. Consequently some attention is freed from the body and the above somatics have not particularly reoccurred in the two years since finishing the program. From my viewpoint as a physician, this raises several questions on what effects low-grade radiation of different types over a lifetime can have on a being or his body—probably more significant than is currently recognized. G.D.

One individual worked on a contamination clean-up crew at the atomic research center in Hanford, Washington. He had worked inside nuclear reactors[8] and once reported inhaling highly contaminated dust. He said he recalled working in one specific area that was so "hot"[9] he was only permitted one minute of work in the area per day. Other areas he'd worked in had longer "burn-out" time such as ten minutes or thirty minutes. He later underwent the Purification program.

---

8. **nuclear reactors:** apparatuses in which an atomic fission chain reaction can be initiated, sustained and controlled, for generating heat or producing useful radiation.

9. **hot:** of, pertaining to or noting radioactivity.

Before the program I felt "massy" around the head. I thought I was doing okay but I knew it wasn't quite right. I felt as though something needed to be handled. While doing the program I went through periods of blankness for days. I just couldn't seem to remember things. Also, I went through about one week of not being able to catch my breath. You know, I didn't even realize I had had a problem with it, but now I can recall shortness of breath while mountain climbing, but only when the weather was hot. After the program, I am in great shape. I feel sharp, alert and ready to face life. I sure do feel better about life and myself now. B.H.

Two particular cases focused on the US atomic testing in the 1950s.

One such case involves a person who grew up in Utah and as a child was exposed to the radioactive fallout from the US government's nuclear tests in neighboring Nevada. He completed the Purification program in February of 1980 and described some of his experiences:

It should be noted what happened one night in the sauna. After I had been in there for some three hours I turned on a tremendous amount of radiation. There was no redness with the niacin, merely the tremendous heat and pain I felt when I got a good deal of radiation from atomic blasts in 1953. I almost died from radiation burns at that time. I received a great deal of atomic radiation from drinking water that had been filled with fallout. In the sauna I experienced the full return of that moment. I felt the grief and the anger and the pain and the swelling of the face and the blisters and the pain through to the bones. I then went back into the sauna and was able to "blow off" a good deal of this feeling by further sauna exposure.

I feel I have now run out all the drugs and the extreme radiation that I was exposed to in this life-time. I regained my affinity for people and have a greater love and tolerance for them as a result of the drugs being removed. There have been times on this program when I felt such exhilaration and felt the way I felt when I was a kid . . . My energy level has picked up tremendously.

My friends that I grew up with have not been so fortunate. The atomic tests or the fallout from those tests in Nevada, falling on Utah, have done such a great deal of damage to so many lives. Some of my friends in Utah are dead as a result of those tests. My life would have gone by the boards[10] if I had not had this program. There is a deep sense of gratitude to L. Ron Hubbard for this program. H.J.

Another case was a man who was one of 2,100 marines who received orders to participate in nuclear weapons testing at the Nevada test site. He witnessed two atomic detonations in June and July of 1957. The second explosion, 77 kilotons,[11] was the largest atmospheric blast test ever conducted within the continental limits of the United States. He was in an open trench 3 miles from the explosion. Shortly afterwards, he was

---

10. **gone by the boards:** literally, gone over the ship's side, from the nautical definition of *boards* meaning "the sides of a ship." Used figuratively, it means "been destroyed, neglected or forgotten."

11. **kilotons:** measurements of explosive force equal to that of 1,000 tons of TNT.

sent in to within 300 yards of "ground zero."[12] He once described to a newspaper reporter his recollection of the first blast.

> We were told to bend down in the ditch and cover our eyes with our forearms. When that blast went off, I could see the bone in my arm through my closed eyes . . . We were thrown back and forth in that ditch. It was like a stampede of cattle went over us. The force and heat were tremendous. We had burns on the back of our necks. We weren't prepared ahead of time for any of this . . . We were as innocent as children until that bomb lit up the sky as bright as day and I turned to see a manikin[13] behind me with its face on fire.

In 1978, he started feeling sick. He said he went to thirty-six doctors but they couldn't determine what was wrong with him. Years later people had told him about the program and in 1983 he decided to try it. He reported his observations:

> My improvements were multifaceted.[14] When I began this program I had reached the point where I felt that a return to well-being was highly improbable if not impossible. During the first thirteen to fourteen days of the program I continued to believe that improvement was out of the question for me. And then— WHAMO! Something miraculous happened! Damned if I didn't begin to feel better. A little better at first in subtle yet noticeable ways. For instance, my stamina increased; my feelings of tiredness began to

---

12. **ground zero:** the point on the surface of the earth or water directly below, directly above or at which an atomic or hydrogen bomb explodes.

13. **manikin:** a model of the human body for teaching anatomy, demonstrating surgical operations, etc.

14. **multifaceted:** having many aspects or phases.

dissipate slowly and grudgingly. Towards the end of the program I realized that I had more vitality than at any time in the last seven or eight years. Emotionally, I felt up. Depression lifted and I could once again feel exhilaration when such moments occurred. There is new hope for radiation victims! I'm the living proof of it! T.S.

Chemical Exposure: An Occupational Case History

One which was particularly noteworthy involved a woman who went to her physician complaining of chemical exposure. Among her complaints were a constant feeling of tiredness, skin problems, and a general feeling of "feeling terrible all the time." She said she was exposed to toxic chemicals during her employment at an electronics manufacturing company. Each night she cleaned filters in a system designed to entrap soot and other particles. She washed them with already contaminated water which she described as blackish and oily.

After several interviews with medical experts, an occupational health specialist suggested she undergo L. Ron Hubbard's program under his care. She decided to do so.

Four days into the program she reported "black junk" coming from her pores that resembled water she used at work. This was noted on the arms, neck, face. The outpouring of this black, oily material continued throughout the program though in lesser and lesser amounts until she was done.

Her physician, a diplomate[15] in occupational medicine and

---

15. **diplomate:** a person who has received a diploma, especially a doctor, engineer, etc., who has been certified as a specialist by a board within the appropriate profession.

a medical doctor for over twenty years, who also holds a Masters of Public Health degree, reported his observations which included the following:

> I saw her for a post-treatment evaluation. Subjectively, she was feeling fine . . . She noted specifically a great increase in her energy level, felt that her eyesight was much improved, that her skin had cleared considerably, including improvement in the gum problems that she had noted, hair less oily, and other subjective improvements such as better outlook on life, decrease in the lymph gland[16] swellings, and a general improvement in her feeling of well-being. . . .

> In summary, [this patient] has had a very successful response to the Hubbard program of detoxification. She feels well and is ready to return to full employment of any type which she can find.

> I am convinced that the Hubbard program of detoxification is the only mechanism now available to rid the body of fat-soluble toxic substances. I believe this case will amply demonstrate that it is, indeed, effective.

Agent Orange: Case Histories

In the last several years, one of the most controversial if not explosive toxic contamination topics has been Agent Orange,

---

16. **lymph gland:** any of the glandlike masses of tissue in the body which create *lymph*, a clear, yellowish fluid containing white blood cells in a liquid resembling blood plasma.

the herbicide-defoliant sprayed by United States military aircraft in the jungles of Vietnam. The key ingredient in Agent Orange is dioxin, a deadly chemical reported to store in body tissues and which even in minute quantities can cause serious adverse health effects.

There have been several cases where individuals who claimed they had been exposed to Agent Orange completed the Purification program. While no facility delivering the Purification program makes claims for the elimination of Agent Orange symptoms, the following reports are examples that do offer great hope.

> *Prior to the Purification program something was wrong. Objectively, I was acting analytically but from time to time subjectively I would experience psychosis and neurosis in specific areas of my life which tended to hamper me as a being. I am an ex-Marine who had fought in the Vietnam War from 1968 to 1969.*
>
> *Besides the constant fighting, I also was exposed to deadly poisonous gases and toxins, especially Agent Orange and some sort of nerve gas, while in the service and in the Vietnam War. Through the Purification program these toxins were fully flushed out. They had actually prevented me from thinking straight and logically; inhibited my perceptions and control of my body. Boy, was I ever in for a surprise during the program and after completion!*
>
> *I literally erased an incident which had me stuck on "the track,"[17] dramatizing it in present time, that I*

---

17. **track:** short for *time track*. See **time track** in the glossary.

wasn't aware of. I had considered my environment dangerous—I mean really dangerous, as it was in the jungles of South Vietnam. But would you believe that I was still "in" South Vietnam though I left it in 1969? I was fully brought out of it as well as oriented to my present environment by the Purification program.

It really undercut[18] everything. I mean, these were such very simple actions to do but powerful insofar as the results and gains I had. Both objectively and subjectively, the Purification program has changed my life, my physical well-being and my attitude towards a much better existence of survival. I no longer have to look over my shoulder for "the enemy" (which wasn't there) or walk carefully through any grassy areas (looking for land mines which don't exist) so that I can live another day.

It has opened a door for me—a door through which I can experience life. My physical being is much better insofar as its coloration and pigment. Many other people have commented on how healthy I look. I feel healthy and I am aware that I am in control of my body which had been hampered prior to the Purification program by those toxins, especially Agent Orange. As a Vietnam vet, I can say that life is definitely worthwhile to experience and create. There is hope for those Vietnam vets who are still in the Vietnam War syndrome after being out of the war. W.B.

---

18. **undercut:** literally, to cut under or beneath. Used figuratively to describe the action of handling something very basic or fundamental, which then allows one to handle more complex problems or aspects of something.

Here is another report, from a man who enlisted in the Army in 1962. In 1964, he was airlifted to Saigon, Vietnam, and from there on to Thailand.[19] In a legally sworn affidavit, he tells his story:

During that year, October 1964 to October 1965, I noticed that aircraft would sometimes spray the jungle just outside the base I was on. During one of these sprayings the wind was blowing in my direction and some of the spray mist landed on my skin in the area of my neck and upper chest. A corporal had told me that the spraying was done to keep the jungle from growing too high. Within a week or so of the spray coming in contact with my skin, I had developed open sores that bled slightly. These were just in the area that the spray mist had touched.

I went to the field hospital to have this condition checked as I was afraid of what was happening. These sores did not heal at all and seemed to be getting worse. I was examined at that field hospital and the sores were diagnosed as acne;[20] very acute acne. I was told to wash better and was given some peroxide[21] to use to clean the sores. I did exactly as told and the sores got deeper. One was so deep that I could put a "Q-Tip"[22] all the way into it and past the

---

19. **Thailand:** a kingdom in Southeast Asia, formerly called Siam.

20. **acne:** a common skin disease, especially among young people, in which the oil-secreting glands in the skin become inflamed and cause pimples on the face, back and chest.

21. **peroxide:** hydrogen peroxide; a colorless liquid used in a diluted solution as a bleach and an antiseptic.

22. **Q-Tip:** (*trademark*) a brand of cotton-tipped swab used especially for cleansing a small area or for applying medications or cosmetics.

cotton swab on the end of the "Q-Tip." I must say I felt very apathetic about this condition.

I was due for return to the United States and release from the service in October 1965. I went again to the field hospital for my medical release and again was told I did not wash good enough and still had the acne. I was not and am not a doctor so I believed what I was told and took my release and returned to the United States where I was discharged.

From October 1965 until sometime in 1978 I had these sores. They were always open and sometimes bleeding slightly. Sometimes I would also be upset mentally.

During 1978 I was a parishioner at the Church of Scientology Mission of Fort Lauderdale, Florida. One of the services offered at the mission at the time was a program designed to handle the harmful effects of drug residues stored in the body. This program was called the "Sweat Program."

Within two weeks after starting the "Sweat Program" besides the spiritual benefit I was feeling, the sores had cleared up and I felt good again although the sores had not totally disappeared.

The "Sweat Program" was later refined and improved upon and was replaced by the Purification program. During 1981 I did the Purification program and the sores healed totally. It was while on this program that

I finally realized that the sores came from the Agent Orange that I was exposed to in 1965.

The experience related above was not unique. Another man served with a Marine Air Traffic Control Unit in Vietnam from August 1967 to August 1968. He was sure he was exposed to Agent Orange as they sprayed the defoliant within two or three miles of his base.

Upon returning from Vietnam, I had continual problems with rashes all over my body. I later found out this is termed chloracne.[23] I also had liver problems, continuous headaches (migraines[24]) and an inability to tolerate much liquor without getting ill. Additionally, my wife had two miscarriages and had since not been able to get pregnant.

About a year ago, I completed the Purification program. I no longer am troubled with the chloracne. I still have white spots on my body where I had had rashes in the past. I seldom have headaches and the headaches I do have are rarely of the intensity of the ones I previously had.

My wife is now pregnant again and is over four months along. The longest she was able to carry a pregnancy in the past was less than three months. I attribute these changes in my physical health directly to having done L. Ron Hubbard's Purification program.

---

23. **chloracne:** a severe and sometimes persistent form of acne resulting from exposure to chlorine compounds, such as dioxin. *See also* **acne** and **dioxin** in the glossary.

24. **migraines:** intense, periodically returning headaches, usually limited to one side of the head and often accompanied by nausea, visual disorders, etc.

This ex-Marine wrote his report in December of 1981. The child he was expecting at the time was born healthy, a baby boy. And his family has grown since then, as the couple went on to have another child, a healthy baby girl.

Scientific Testing

Three years after the program was released, it was independently tested on a group of people who were contaminated with a fire-retardant chemical (polybrominated biphenyls or PBBs).* They were residents of the state of Michigan where millions of people were exposed to the chemical during a massive agricultural contamination in the early 1970s. Previous studies had already established that it takes ten to twenty years or more for the stored residues of PBBs and similar chemicals, such as PCBs (polychlorinated biphenyls, components which are found in industrial coolants) to be reduced naturally by just one half. In light of this, the group of researchers designed a study to measure their fat levels of PBBs, PCBs and several other chemicals before, immediately after, and four months following Purification program. The results were quite startling.

---

* In the summer of 1973, toxic fire-retardant chemicals were accidentally added to livestock feed in Michigan. An extensive study by researchers from Mount Sinai School of Medicine in New York City indicated that even five years after the accident, nearly all of the state's population had been contaminated with polybrominated biphenyls or PBBs. The contamination incident is detailed in several publications. Some suggested ones include: *PBB: An American Tragedy*, by Erwin Chen, Prentice-Hall, 1979; *The Contamination Crisis in Michigan: Polybrominated Biphenyls, A Report From The Senate Special Investigation Committee*, Michigan State Senate, July 1975.

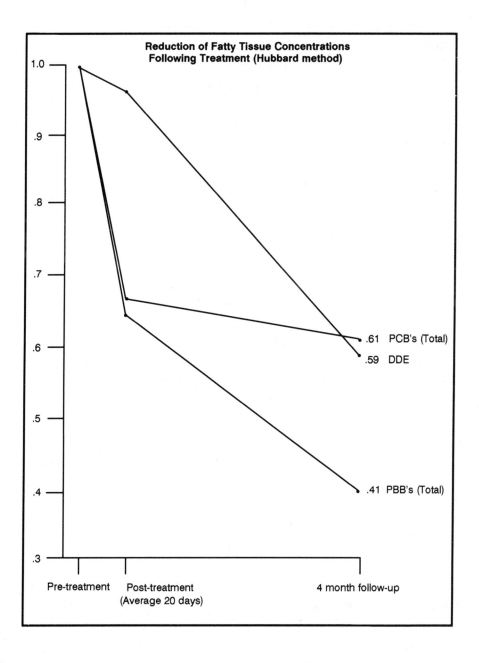

Reduction of Fatty Tissue Concentrations
Following Treatment (Hubbard method)

.61 PCB's (Total)

.59 DDE

.41 PBB's (Total)

Pre-treatment   Post-treatment   4 month follow-up
                 (Average 20 days)

Reduction of Toxic Chemical Levels in the Body

The study group reported that the Purification program brought about an immediate average reduction of approximately 20 percent for 16 different chemicals studied. The results of a four-month follow-up examination revealed an average reduction of over 40 percent for all chemicals. The fact that the chemical levels continued to go down after the program was completed was a phenomenon found in other studies as well. In 1984, a physician reported in the journal, *Clinical Research,* his findings after testing the fat of a person who underwent the program. At the end of 53 days, he reported that the tissue level of a DDT-related chemical (DDE) was reduced by 29 percent. At the end of 250 days—long after his patient had completed the Purification program—the DDE level had been reduced by 97 percent.

Writing in the May 1984 magazine of the US National Safety Council, researcher Dr. Max Ben said, "Given the fact that more than 20 million Americans work with chemicals known to be toxic to the nervous system and other parts of the body, the potential benefits of detoxification techniques such as that developed by Hubbard are immense. If, as the Hubbard regimen seems to indicate, chemical toxins can be removed safely and effectively from the body, then it may be possible to resolve the entire problem of human contamination and chemically related disease."

Conclusion

The editors' intention in this appendix has been to offer not promises of cures or claims but a relative handful of examples of what thousands of people have experienced when undergoing the Purification program as described in this book. It would not be difficult to fill an entire book with such reports—the benefits people report cover an enormous range of improvement categories. We have attempted to select those case reports which would provide a broad view of the type of persons who undergo the program and the types of phenomena which have been reported.

The Editors

Appendix B

Where to Do the Purification Program

Churches have existed since the dawn of man with the purpose of assisting people in their aspirations toward happier and more fulfilling lives.

With the escalation of the drug problem and its disastrous consequences both for the individual and the society, offering a service which can help a person overcome and reverse the damage caused by drugs and toxins becomes a vital necessity to fulfilling such a purpose.

Since 1980, Churches of Scientology have been offering just such a service—L. Ron Hubbard's Purification program. Tens of thousands of people have successfully completed the program at Scientology churches and organizations. The statements of those who have finished the program are full of wonder at the improvements in themselves and praise for the man who researched and developed the program—L. Ron Hubbard.

Mr. Hubbard's life's work was devoted to developing a technology with which to help people attain spiritual awareness and freedom. As he said in an article called *My Philosophy:*

> "I like to help others and count it as my greatest pleasure in life to see a person free himself of the shadows which darken his days.
>
> "These shadows look so thick to him, and weigh him down so, that when he finds they *are* shadows and that he can see through them, walk through them and be again in the sun, he is enormously delighted. And I am afraid that I am just as delighted as he is."

There is no reason for *anyone* to be trapped in the shadows of the effects of drugs and toxins.

Scientology churches and organizations are fully set up to deliver the Purification program, with technical personnel thoroughly trained in the exact application and supervision of the program. Every day, people walk into Scientology organizations around the world and start the Purification program. These are people from all walks of life: former drug addicts, businessmen, celebrities, housewives. Their reasons for starting the program differ, but in doing the program each one is taking a major step on the road to true freedom and personal ability.

You can do the Purification program at a Scientology church or organization in your own area. A list of Scientology organizations is included at the back of this book—contact the one nearest you.

The Purification program provides a means by which an individual, a group and a whole society might take the first step up toward a toxin-free, drug-free civilization.

It is offered here as an invitation to start living!

The Editors

About the Author

About the Author

L. Ron Hubbard is one of the most acclaimed and widely read authors of all time, primarily because his works express a firsthand knowledge of the nature of man—knowledge gained not from standing on the sidelines but through lifelong experience with people from all walks of life.

As Ron said, "One doesn't learn about life by sitting in an ivory tower, thinking about it. One learns about life by being part of it." And that is how he lived.

He began his quest for knowledge on the nature of man at a very early age. When he was eight years old he was already well on his way to being a seasoned traveler. His adventures included voyages to China, Japan and other points in the Orient and South Pacific, covering a quarter of a million miles by the age of nineteen. In the course of his travels he became closely acquainted with twenty-one different races and cultures all over the world.

In the fall of 1930, Ron pursued his studies of mathematics and engineering, enrolling at George Washington University where he was also a member of one of the first American classes on nuclear physics. He realized that neither the East nor the West contained the full answer to the problems of existence.

Despite all of mankind's advances in the physical sciences, a *workable* technology of the mind and life had never been developed. The mental "technologies" which did exist, psychology and psychiatry, were actually barbaric, false subjects—no more workable than the methods of jungle witch doctors. Ron shouldered the responsibility of filling this gap in the knowledge of mankind.

He financed his early research through fiction writing. He became one of the most highly demanded authors in the golden age of popular adventure and science fiction writing during the 1930s and 1940s, interrupted only by his service in the US Navy during World War II.

Partially disabled at the war's end, Ron applied what he had learned from his researches. He made breakthroughs and developed techniques which made it possible for him to recover from his injuries and help others to regain their health. It was during this time that the basic tenets of Dianetics technology were codified. Part of his early research into the nature of mental phenomena included a study of the endocrine system and effect of the mind on the body's ability to absorb and use nutrients.

In 1948, he wrote a manuscript detailing his discoveries. It was not published at that time, but circulated amongst Ron's friends, who copied it and passed it on to others. (This manuscript was formally published in 1951 as *Dianetics: The Original Thesis* and later republished as *The Dynamics of Life*.) The interest generated by this manuscript prompted a flood of requests for more information on the subject.

Ron provided all his discoveries to the American Psychiatric Association and the American Medical Association. Despite the fact that his work would have benefited them and society immensely, they ignored his research and continued on with their archaic activities.

Meanwhile, the steadily increasing flow of letters asking for further information and requesting that he detail more applications of his new subject resulted in Ron spending all his time answering letters. He decided to write and publish a comprehensive text on the subject—*Dianetics: The Modern Science of Mental Health.*

With the release of *Dianetics* on 9 May 1950, a complete handbook for the application of Ron's new technology was broadly available for the first time. Public interest spread like wildfire. The book shot to the top of the *New York Times* best-seller list and remained there week after week. More than 750 Dianetics study groups sprang up within a few months of its publication.

Ron's work did not stop with the success of *Dianetics* but accelerated, with new discoveries and breakthroughs a constant, normal occurrence. In his further research he discovered the very nature of life itself and its exact relationship to this universe. These discoveries led to his development of Scientology, the first workable technology for the improvement of conditions in any aspect of life.

One of the areas Ron gave special attention to in his work was drug rehabilitation. He developed technology, now in use by Narconon centers, which makes it possible for hard-core drug users to recover fully from their addictions. Using his techniques exclusively, Narconon centers have an impressive rate of success in helping people to come off drugs—and *stay* off them.

Ron also conducted extensive studies in the fields of vitamins, minerals and nutrition, resulting in breakthroughs which helped addicts come off drugs more easily, without having to go through the well-known horrors of painful and dangerous withdrawal symptoms.

During the explosion of drug use around the world in the 1960s and early 1970s, he found that people could not achieve the full gains possible from Dianetics and Scientology techniques unless the effects caused by drugs were relieved. He developed techniques to handle the mental effects of drugs, and in further research discovered the factor of drug residuals lodging in the body. From this discovery the Purification program was developed, which Ron released in 1979.

Ron continued his research and writing through 1985, amassing an enormous volume of material totaling over 60 million words—recorded in books, manuscripts and taped lectures. Today these works are studied and applied daily in hundreds of Scientology churches, missions and organizations around the world.

With his research fully completed and codified, L. Ron Hubbard departed his body on 24 January 1986.

Ron opened a wide bridge to understanding and freedom for mankind. Through his efforts, there now exists a totally workable technology with which people can help each other improve their lives and succeed in achieving their goals.

Glossary

acne: a common skin disease, especially among young people, in which the oil-secreting glands in the skin become inflamed and cause pimples on the face, back and chest.

adage: a traditional saying expressing a common experience or observation; proverb.

additive: a thing which has been added. This usually has a bad meaning in that an *additive* is said to be something needless or harmful which has been done in addition to standard procedure. *Additive* normally means a departure from standard procedure. For example, someone administering the Purification program puts different or additional nutritional requirements into the basic lineup called for by the program. It means a twist on standard procedure. In common English, *additive* might mean a substance put into a compound to improve its qualities or suppress undesirable qualities. In this book it definitely means to add something to the technical procedure resulting in undesirable results.

Agent Orange: a powerful herbicide and defoliant containing trace amounts of dioxin, a toxic impurity suspected of causing serious health problems, including cancer and genetic damage, in some persons exposed to it, and birth defects in their offspring; used by US armed forces during the Vietnam War to defoliate jungles (1965–70). The name *Agent Orange* came from the color of the identifying stripe on the drums in which it was stored. *See also* **dioxin** and **defoliant** in this glossary.

algae: a group of plants, either one-celled or many-celled, often growing in colonies. Algae contain chlorophyll (the green coloring matter of plants) and other pigments, but have no true root, stem or leaf. They are found in water or damp places and include seaweed, pond scum, etc.

alkaline: of or like the class of substances that neutralize and are neutralized by acids, and form caustic or corrosive solutions in water.

amino acids: basic organic compounds which are essential to the body's breakdown and absorption of foods.

anemic: suffering from *anemia,* a condition in which there is a reduction of the number, or volume, of red blood cells or of the total amount of hemoglobin (the oxygen-carrying pigment of red blood cells that gives them their red color and serves to convey oxygen to the tissues) in the bloodstream, resulting in paleness, generalized weakness, etc.

angel dust: (*slang*) phencyclidine, an anesthetic drug used as an animal tranquilizer; also widely used in several forms as an illicit hallucinogen. Also called *PCP.*

asbestos: any of several grayish minerals that separate into long, threadlike fibers. Because certain varieties do not burn, do not conduct heat or electricity and are often resistant to chemicals, they are used for making fireproof materials, electrical insulation, roofing, filters, etc. Known to cause lung cancer when inhaled.

atrophy: a wasting away of the body or of an organ or part, as from defective nutrition or nerve damage.

autopsies: inspections and dissections of bodies after death, as for determination of the cause of death; post-mortem examinations.

B$_1$: *see* **vitamin B$_1$.**

B$_2$: *see* **vitamin B$_2$.**

B$_6$: *see* **vitamin B$_6$.**

B$_{12}$: *see* **vitamin B$_{12}$.**

bacterial: caused by *bacteria*, typically one-celled organisms which can be seen only with a microscope. They occur in three main forms—spherical, rod-shaped and spiral; some bacteria cause diseases such as pneumonia and tuberculosis, and others are necessary for fermentation, decomposition, etc.

B complex: *see* **vitamin B complex.**

bioplasma: a dietary supplement taken to replenish depleted supplies of various mineral salts naturally found in the body.

biotin: a vitamin important in protein, carbohydrate and unsaturated fatty acid metabolism, normal growth and maintenance of skin, hair, nerves, bone marrow and various glands.

bird: a person, especially one having some peculiarity.

boards, gone by the: literally, gone over the ship's side, from the nautical definition of *boards* meaning "the sides of a ship." Used figuratively, it means "been destroyed, neglected or forgotten."

bomb, works like a: does something extremely well.

borne out: substantiated; confirmed.

brief (hold a brief for): support or defend by argument; endorse.

bronchial: of or pertaining to the bronchi (the major passageways of the lungs; especially either of the two main branches of the trachea, or windpipe) and their smaller subdivisions.

cadavers: dead bodies, especially human bodies to be dissected; corpses.

catalytic: causing or accelerating a chemical change without itself (the substance causing the change) being affected.

centigrade: pertaining to or noting a temperature scale in which 0 degrees represents the ice point and 100 degrees the steam point. Also called *Celsius.*

chelated: a process by which minerals are held, as if by a claw, by amino acids. *Chelation* is taken from a Greek word meaning "claw." This bonding of a mineral with an amino acid exists in nature as a necessary step for the mineral to be absorbed and used by the body. Thus, with this step already provided, the mineral is more easily absorbed and used. *See also* **amino acids** in this glossary.

chicken out: stop doing something because of fear; decide not to do something after all even though previously having decided to try it.

chloracne: a severe and sometimes persistent form of acne resulting from exposure to chlorine compounds, such as dioxin. *See also* **acne** and **dioxin** in this glossary.

choline: a vitamin important to the functioning of the nervous system (it is an essential ingredient in the nerve fluid), the liver and the buildup of immunities.

cinch: (*slang*) something that is sure to happen or easy to do.

coal tar: a thick, black, sticky liquid formed during the distillation of coal, that upon further distillation yields compounds from which are derived a large number of dyes, drugs and other synthetic compounds.

cocaine: a bitter, crystalline drug obtained from the dried leaves of the coca shrub; it is a local anesthetic and a dangerous, illegal stimulant.

codeine: a narcotic derived from opium and resembling morphine, but less habit-forming: used for the relief of pain and in cough medicines.

cold-pressed: produced through extraction by pressure without the use of heat.

cold turkey: (*slang*) abrupt and complete withdrawal from the use of an addictive substance, as a narcotic drug, alcohol or tobacco.

colitis: inflammation of the colon (a part of the large intestine).

considerations: thoughts or beliefs about something.

cords: tendons: any of the inelastic cords of tough, fibrous connective tissue in which muscle fibers end and by which muscles are attached to bones or other parts; sinews.

curtail: cut short; reduce; abridge.

Davis, Adelle: prominent American nutritionist, author of books on nutrition, including *Let's Eat Right to Keep Fit, Let's Cook It Right, Let's Have Healthy Children* and *Let's Get Well.*

debilitated: reduced to *debility,* the condition of being weak or feeble; weak intellectually or morally.

debility: weakness or feebleness, especially of the body.

defoliant: a chemical used to destroy or cause widespread loss of leaves, as in an area of jungle, forest, etc., used to deprive enemy troops or guerrilla forces of concealment.

deity: a god or goddess.

delirium tremens: a violent delirium (temporary state of extreme mental excitement, marked by restlessness, confused speech and hallucinations) resulting chiefly from excessive drinking of alcoholic liquor and characterized by sweating, trembling, anxiety and frightening hallucinations. *Delirium tremens* comes from Latin, and means literally "trembling delirium."

demeanor: conduct; behavior.

detoxification: the act of ridding of a poison or the effect of a poison.

dexterity: skill or adroitness in using the hands or body; agility; also, mental adroitness or skill; cleverness.

dioxin: a highly toxic chemical that occurs as an impurity in some herbicides and defoliants.

diplomate: a person who has received a diploma, especially a doctor, engineer, etc., who has been certified as a specialist by a board within the appropriate profession.

dispirited: discouraged; dejected; disheartened; gloomy.

dissipating: becoming scattered or dispersed; being dispelled; disintegrating.

DNA: abbreviation for *deoxyribonucleic acid*; a complex compound found in the nucleus of all living cells which plays a vital part in heredity. It is the chief material in chromosomes, the cell bodies that control the heredity of an animal or a plant. The DNA in the chromosomes furnishes the cells with a complete set of "instructions" for their own development and the development of their descendants for generations.

dormant: in a state of rest or inactivity; inoperative.

dramatize: repeat in action what has happened to one in experience; replay now something that happened then. *Dramatization* is the duplication of the content of a mental image picture, entire or in part, by a person in his present time environment. The degree of dramatization is in direct ratio to the degree of restimulation of the mental image pictures causing it. When dramatizing, the individual is like an actor playing his dictated part and going through a whole series of irrational actions. *See also* **mental image picture** and **restimulation** in this glossary.

efficacy: capacity for producing a desired result or effect; effectiveness.

electrons: any of the negatively charged particles that form a part of all atoms, and can exist on their own in a free state.

embedded: having become fixed or incorporated, as into a surrounding mass.

empirical: derived from or guided by experience or experiment.

encumbered: impeded or hindered; hampered.

endocrine system: the system of glands which produce one or more internal secretions that, introduced directly into the bloodstream, are carried to other parts of the body whose functions they regulate or control.

enzymes: complex organic substances secreted by certain cells of plants and animals which cause a chemical change in the substance upon which they act.

epidemic: extremely prevalent; widespread.

ether: a drug used to produce anesthesia, as before surgery.

eucalyptus: any of numerous often tall trees native to Australia and adjacent islands, having aromatic evergreen leaves that are the source of medicinal oils and heavy wood used as timber.

euthanasia: the original definition of *euthanasia* is "mercy killing," the act of putting to death painlessly or allowing to die (as by withholding extreme medical measures) a person or animal suffering from an incurable disease or condition. However, under the practice of psychiatry it has become "the act of killing people considered a burden on society."

exudation: the action of coming out gradually in drops, as sweat, through pores or small openings; oozing out.

faddism: the practice of following a fad (a temporary fashion, notion, manner of conduct, etc., especially one followed enthusiastically by a group), such as seeking and adhering briefly to a passing variety of unusual diets, beliefs, etc.

fallout: the descent to earth of radioactive particles, as after a nuclear explosion or reactor accident; also the radioactive particles themselves.

fasting: abstaining from all food.

fatty tissues: tissues (substances of an organic body or organ, made up of cells and the material between them) which contain or consist of fat.

fiber: the structural part of plants and plant products that consists of carbohydrates that are wholly or partially indigestible and when eaten helps to move waste products through the intestines.

flare up: begin again suddenly, especially for a short time after a quiet time.

flush: the reddening of the skin caused by a rush of blood; also, the rush of blood itself.

folic acid: a vitamin important in the formation of red blood cells.

full-blown: fully developed; complete.

gastroenteritis: an inflammation of the stomach and the intestines.

genesis: the way in which something comes to be; beginning; origin.

ginseng: any of several plants of eastern Asia or North America having an aromatic root used medicinally.

gout: an acute, recurrent disease characterized by painful inflammation of the joints, chiefly those in the feet and hands, and especially in the big toe, and by an excess of uric acid (a white, odorless substance found in urine) in the blood.

gradient: a gradual approach to something taken step by step, level by level, each step or level being, of itself, easily surmountable—so that finally, quite complicated and difficult activities can be achieved with relative ease.

ground zero: the point on the surface of the earth or water directly below, directly above or at which an atomic or hydrogen bomb explodes.

hallucinogen: a drug or other substance that produces hallucinations.

harboring: keeping or holding in the mind; maintaining; entertaining.

hashish: a drug made from the resin contained in the flowering tops of hemp, chewed or smoked for its intoxicating and euphoric effects.

heat exhaustion: a condition characterized by faintness, rapid pulse, nausea, profuse sweating, cool skin and collapse, caused by prolonged exposure to heat accompanied by loss of adequate fluid and salt from the body.

heatstroke: a disturbance of the temperature-regulating mechanisms of the body caused by overexposure to excessive heat, resulting in fever, hot and dry skin and rapid pulse, sometimes progressing to delirium and coma.

heretofore: before this time; until now.

heroin: a white, crystalline, narcotic powder, derived from morphine, formerly used as a painkiller and sedative; manufacture and importation of heroin is controlled by federal law in the US because of the danger of addiction. The word is derived from the Greek word *hero* allegedly because of the feelings of power and euphoria which it stimulates.

hives: a disease in which the skin itches and shows raised, white welts, caused by a sensitivity to certain foods or a reaction to heat, light, etc.

hobbyhorsing: concerning oneself excessively with a favorite notion or activity; variation of the phrase *ride a hobbyhorse.*

hot: of, pertaining to or noting radioactivity.

hung-over: of or pertaining to the disagreeable physical after-effects of drunkenness, such as a headache or stomach disorder, usually felt several hours after cessation of drinking.

hypnotics: agents or drugs that produce sleep; sedatives.

impinge: make an impression; have an effect or impact.

impregnated: infused or permeated throughout, as with a substance; saturated.

indicator: a condition or circumstance arising during an action which indicates whether the action is running well or badly. A bad condition not getting any better or not lessening, or the person having losses would be *bad indicators.* A bad condition getting better or becoming less present would be a *good indicator. Good indicators* also include such things as fast progress, person happy, having wins, etc.

inositol: a vitamin found in high concentrations in the human brain, stomach, kidney, spleen and liver; related to control of cholesterol level; reported to have mild inhibitory effect on cancer.

iodine: a chemical element found in seawater and certain seaweeds, used in solution as an antiseptic; iodine is used by the thyroid gland (a large gland at the front of the neck, secreting a hormone that regulates the body's growth and development) to help regulate metabolism, and a shortage of iodine can cause goiter (enlargement of the thyroid gland).

ion: an electrically charged atom or group of atoms formed by the loss or gain of one or more electrons. A positive ion is created by electron loss, and a negative ion is created by electron gain.

IU: abbreviation for *international unit*, an internationally agreed-upon standard to which samples of a substance, as a drug or hormone, are compared to ascertain their relative potency. *IU* also stands for the particular quantity of such a substance which causes a specific biological effect.

kick: an intense, personal, usually temporary, preference, habit or passion; a fad.

kicks: thrills; pleasurable excitement.

kilotons: measurements of explosive force equal to that of 1,000 tons of TNT.

lamentable: deplorable; regrettable.

lecithin: a complex fatty substance which is found in egg yolk and contains phosphorus (a mineral which helps give strength to bones and aids in metabolism).

letdown: a decrease in energy, force, volume, etc.

Librium: trademark for a tranquilizing drug, used by psychiatrists in an attempt to suppress the symptoms of anxiety.

loaded: (*slang*) under the influence of alcohol or drugs.

LSD: a crystalline solid substance which is a powerful psychedelic drug, producing temporary hallucinations and a schizophrenic psychotic state. *LSD* is an abbreviation for *lysergic acid diethylamide*.

lucid: characterized by clear perception or understanding; rational or sane.

lymph gland: any of the glandlike masses of tissue in the body which create *lymph,* a clear, yellowish fluid containing white blood cells in a liquid resembling blood plasma.

manganese: a mineral important to growth, bone formation, reproduction, muscle coordination and fat and carbohydrate metabolism.

manifestations: outward or perceptible indications; materializations.

manikin: a model of the human body for teaching anatomy, demonstrating surgical operations, etc.

marijuana: the dried leaves and flowers of the hemp plant, used in cigarette form as a narcotic or hallucinogen.

marrow: a soft fatty tissue in the interior cavities of bones that is a major site of blood cell production.

megavitamin: of, pertaining to or using very large amounts of vitamins.

mental image pictures: mental copies of one's perceptions sometime in the past; three-dimensional color pictures with sound and smell and all other perceptions, plus the conclusions or speculations of the individual. For example, a person who had taken LSD would retain "pictures" of that experience in his mind, complete with recordings of the sights, physical sensations, smells, sounds, etc., that occurred while he was under the influence of LSD. For further information on mental image pictures and how the mind works, read the book *Dianetics: The Modern Science of Mental Health* by L. Ron Hubbard.

metabolism: the sum of the physical and chemical processes in an organism by which its material substance is produced, maintained and destroyed, and by which energy is made available.

methadone: a synthetic narcotic, similar to morphine but effective orally, used in the relief of pain and as a heroin substitute in the treatment of heroin addiction. Methadone failed as a "solution" to heroin addiction because people instead became addicted to methadone.

migraines: intense, periodically returning headaches, usually limited to one side of the head and often accompanied by nausea, visual disorders, etc.

misemotion: a coined word that is used to mean an emotion or emotional reaction that is inappropriate to the present time situation. It is taken from *mis-* (wrong) + *emotion.* To say that a person was *misemotional* would indicate that the person did not display the emotion called for by the actual circumstances of the situation. Being misemotional would be synonymous with being irrational. One can fairly judge the rationality of any individual by the correctness of the emotion he displays in a given set of circumstances. To be joyful and happy when circumstances call for joy and happiness would be rational. To display grief without sufficient present time cause would be irrational.

multifaceted: having many aspects or phases.

Narconon: a drug rehabilitation program using L. Ron Hubbard's technology. It was originally organized in the Arizona State Prison by an inmate who was himself a drug addict of thirteen years. He put to use the basic principles of the mind contained in books by L. Ron Hubbard, and by doing so completely cured himself and helped twenty other inmates do the same. *Narconon* means *non-narcosis,* and there are now Narconon centers in many areas around the world. On the Narconon program, no drugs whatever are used for withdrawal, and the usual withdrawal effects, such as those experienced by quitting drugs "cold turkey," are most often completely bypassed.

narcotic: of or having the power to produce *narcosis,* a state of stupor or greatly reduced activity produced by a drug.

nervous system: the system of nerves and nerve centers in an animal or human, including the brain, spinal cord, nerves and masses of nerve tissue.

niacin: a white, odorless, crystalline substance found in protein foods or prepared synthetically. It is a member of the vitamin B complex. *See also* **vitamin B complex** in this glossary.

nuclear reactors: apparatuses in which an atomic fission chain reaction can be initiated, sustained and controlled, for generating heat or producing useful radiation.

nucleus: the central part of an atom, composed of protons and neutrons and making up almost all of the mass of the atom: it carries a positive charge.

Objective Processes: counseling procedures which help a person to look or place his attention outward from himself. *Objective* refers to outward things, not the thoughts or feelings of the individual. Objective Processes deal with the real and observable. They call for the person to spot or find something exterior to himself in order to carry out the procedures. Objective Processes locate the person in his environment, establish direct communication, and bring a person to present time, a very important factor in mental and spiritual sanity and ability.

originations: a coined word meaning statements or remarks volunteered by a person concerning himself, his ideas, reactions or difficulties; communications originated by the person himself.

overrun: the condition of continuing an action or a series of actions past the optimum point, or past the point where that action has ceased to produce change.

PABA: an abbreviation for a vitamin called *para-amino-benzoic acid*; important in the metabolism of protein, blood cell formation, stimulation of intestinal bacteria to produce folic acid and utilization of pantothenic acid. *See also* **folic acid** and **pantothenic acid** in this glossary.

palatable: acceptable or agreeable to the sense of taste.

panacea: a supposed remedy, cure or medicine for all diseases or ills; cure-all.

pantothenic acid: an acid found in plant and animal tissues, rice, bran, etc., that is part of the B complex of vitamins and is essential for cell growth.

patent medicines: medicines sold without a prescription in drugstores or by sales representatives, and usually protected by a trademark.

peroxide: hydrogen peroxide; a colorless liquid used in a diluted solution as a bleach and an antiseptic.

peyote: a hallucinogenic drug prepared from the dried, button-like tops of a type of Mexican cactus.

pharmacopoeias: authoritative books containing lists and descriptions of drugs and medicinal products together with the standards established under law for their production, dispensation, use, etc.

phenobarbital: a white crystalline powder used as a sedative and hypnotic.

physical universe: the material universe, which is made up of matter, energy, space and time.

pilots: preliminary or experimental trials or tests.

placenta: an organ that develops in the womb during pregnancy and supplies the fetus with nourishment.

polyunsaturated: a kind of fat or oil that (unlike animal or dairy fats) is not associated with the formation of cholesterol (a fatty substance associated with hardening of the arteries) in the blood.

potassium: a mineral which helps to keep body fluids balanced and is important to the functioning of the nervous system.

precipitation: a being caused to happen before expected, warranted, needed or desired; a bringing on; a hastening.

precognitive: having knowledge of a future event or situation, especially through extrasensory means.

predisposition: the fact or condition of having an inclination or tendency to beforehand; susceptibility.

present time: the time which is now, rather than in the past. It is a term loosely applied to the environment existing in the present. A person said to be "out of present time" would be someone whose attention is fixed on past events to such an extent that he is not fully aware of or in communication with his actual present environment.

procreate: beget or generate (offspring).

proffered: brought or put before a person for acceptance; offered, presented, tendered.

Program Case Supervisor: that person assigned the responsibility of overseeing the delivery of and ensuring the proper and exact application of all aspects of the Purification program to individual *cases*—persons being treated or helped.

propaganda: information, ideas or rumors deliberately widely spread to help or harm a person, group, movement, institution, nation, etc.

psychedelic: of, pertaining to or noting any of various drugs producing a mental state characterized by a profound sense of intensified sensory perception, sometimes accompanied by severe perceptual distortion and hallucinations and by extreme feelings of either euphoria or despair.

psychosomatic: *psycho* refers to mind and *somatic* refers to body; the term *psychosomatic* means the mind making the body ill or illnesses which have been created physically within the body by derangement of the mind.

Q-Tip: (*trademark*) a brand of cotton-tipped swab used especially for cleansing a small area or for applying medications or cosmetics.

rancid: having a rank, unpleasant, stale smell or taste, as through decomposition, especially of fats or oils.

ravaging: causing havoc or ruinous damage.

regimen: a regulated course, as of diet, exercise or manner of living, intended to preserve or restore health or to attain some result.

restimulation: reactivation of a past memory due to similar circumstances in the present approximating circumstances of the past.

riddled: affected in every part; having (something) spread throughout.

RNA: abbreviation for *ribonucleic acid*; one of the compounds found in all living cells; the substance that carries out DNA's instructions for protein production. *See also* **DNA** in this glossary.

runs out: erases; causes to disappear.

rust: a fungus which causes any of several diseases of plants, characterized by reddish, brownish or black blisterlike swellings on the leaves, stems, etc.

schizophrenics: (*psychiatry*) persons who have *schizophrenia*, a major mental disorder typically characterized by a separation of the thought processes and the emotions, a distortion of reality accompanied by delusions and hallucinations, a fragmentation of the personality, motor (involving muscular movement) disturbances, bizarre behavior, etc. The word *schizophrenia* comes from Greek, meaning *split mind*.

Scientology: Scientology philosophy. It is the study and handling of the spirit in relationship to itself, universes and other life. Scientology means *scio*, knowing in the fullest sense of the word and *logos*, study. In itself the word means literally *knowing how to know*. Scientology is a "route," a way, rather than a dissertation or an assertive body of knowledge. Through its drills and studies one may find the truth for himself. The technology is therefore not expounded as something to believe, but something to *do*.

scurvy: a disease resulting from a deficiency of ascorbic acid (vitamin C) in the body, characterized by weakness, anemia, spongy gums, bleeding from the mucous membranes, etc.

sedatives: drugs intended to lessen excitement, nervousness or irritation.

selenium: a trace mineral which helps to keep muscles healthy, protect cells against oxidation and stimulate the manufacture of antibodies.

sodium pentothal: a yellowish-white drug injected intravenously as a general anesthetic and hypnotic.

somatics: physical pains or discomforts of any kind. The word *somatic* means, actually, bodily or physical. Because the word *pain* has in the past led to confusion between physical pain and mental pain, *somatic* is the term used to denote physical pain or discomfort.

soporifics: things that cause sleep, as medicines or drugs.

spaced-out: dazed or stupefied because of the influence of narcotic drugs.

spacey: same as **spaced-out.**

stint: a period of time spent doing something.

straight: (*slang*) free from using narcotics.

street drugs: drugs which are sold or distributed on the streets, rather than by prescription.

Sweat Program: a program developed by L. Ron Hubbard which involved having a person exercise by jogging or running while wearing a rubberized sweat suit to assist in sweating (for the purpose of getting rid of LSD residues lodged in fatty tissue).

tandem: a relationship between two persons or things involving cooperative action, mutual dependence, etc.

tendered: presented for acceptance; offered.

Thailand: a kingdom in Southeast Asia, formerly called Siam.

time track: the consecutive record of mental image pictures which accumulates through a person's life. *See also* **mental image pictures** in this glossary.

touted: described or advertised boastfully; publicized or promoted; praised extravagantly.

trace minerals: minerals that are required in minute quantities for physiological functioning.

track: short for *time track. See* **time track** in this glossary.

tranquilizers: drugs that have a sedative or calming effect without inducing sleep.

traumatic: distressing; emotionally disturbing.

trips: experiences or periods of euphoria, hallucination, etc., induced by a psychedelic drug, especially LSD.

tune, out of: not in proper harmony or accord; unresponsive.

turning on: starting suddenly to affect or show.

undercut: literally, to cut under or beneath. Used figuratively to describe the action of handling something very basic or fundamental, which then allows one to handle more complex problems or aspects of something.

undue: unwarranted; excessive.

Valium: trademark for a drug called diazepam, a tranquilizer that relaxes muscles and prevents or inhibits convulsions. It is addictive and is often prescribed by doctors or psychiatrists to "relieve" anxiety or tension.

Vietnam: a country in Southeast Asia; divided into North Vietnam and South Vietnam during the Vietnam War, but now reunified.

viral: of or caused by a *virus:* a form of matter smaller than any of the bacteria, that can multiply in living cells and cause disease in animals or plants (smallpox, measles, the flu, etc., are caused by viruses).

vitamin A: a vitamin important in bone growth, healthy skin, sexual function and reproduction.

vitamin B_1: a vitamin, also called thiamine, important to the body in the functions of cell oxidation (respiration), growth, carbohydrate metabolism, stimulation and transmission of nerve impulses, etc.

vitamin B_2: also called riboflavin, a vitamin important in the metabolism of protein and in skin, liver and eye health.

vitamin B_6: a vitamin, also called pyridoxine, important as an enzyme activator in protein, carbohydrate and fat metabolism, hormone production (adrenalin and insulin) and antibody production.

vitamin B_{12}: a vitamin important to red blood cell formation, nervous system health, normal growth, carbohydrate metabolism and fertility.

vitamin B complex: an important group of water-soluble vitamins found in liver, yeast, etc., including vitamin B_1, vitamin B_2 and niacin.

vitamin C: also called ascorbic acid; a colorless, crystalline, water-soluble vitamin, found in many foods, especially citrus fruits, vegetables and rose hips and also made synthetically; it is required for proper nutrition and metabolism.

vitamin D: a vitamin which is important in bone health and growth, calcium metabolism, nerve health and regulation of heartbeat.

vitamin E: a vitamin important in keeping oxygen from combining with waste products to form toxic compounds, and in red blood cell health.

vying: competing; contending.

watchword: a word or phrase expressive of a principle or rule of action; slogan.

wholesale: extensive; broadly indiscriminate.

wins: gains or realizations. Also, intending to do something and doing it or intending not to do something and not doing it. For example, if one intends to be able to communicate better with his boss and does so, that is a win. Or if one intends to no longer be shy around girls and accomplishes that, it is a win.

withdrawal symptoms: any of various symptoms, such as profuse sweating, nausea, etc., induced in a person addicted to a drug when he is deprived of that drug.

woodenness: a condition of being without spirit, animation or awareness; being dull or stupid.

X-rays: a form of radiation similar to light but of a shorter wavelength and capable of penetrating solids; used in medicine for study, diagnosis and treatment of certain organic disorders, especially of internal structures of the body.

Index

Books and Tapes
by L. Ron Hubbard

Purification: An Illustrated Answer to Drugs • Presented in a concise, fully illustrated format, this book provides you with an overview of the Purification program. Our society is ridden by abuse of drugs, alcohol and medicine that reduce one's ability to think clearly. This book lays out what can be done about it, in a form which is easy for anyone to read and understand.

Purification Rundown Delivery Manual • This book is a manual which guides a person through the Purification Rundown step by step. It includes all of the needed reports as well as spaces for the person to write his successes and to attest to program completion. This manual makes administering the Purification Rundown simple and *standard*.

All About Radiation • Can the effects of radiation exposure be avoided or reduced? What exactly would happen in the event of an atomic explosion? Get the answers to these and many other questions in this illuminating book. *All About Radiation* describes observations and discoveries concerning the physical and mental effects of radiation and the possibilities for handling them. Get the real facts on the subject of radiation and its effects.

Basic Scientology Books

The Basic Scientology Books Package contains the knowledge you need to be able to improve conditions in life. These books are available individually or as a set, complete with an attractive slipcase.

Scientology: The Fundamentals of Thought • Improve life *and* make a better world with this easy-to-read book that lays out the fundamental truths about life and thought. No such knowledge has ever before existed, and no such results have ever before been attainable as those which can be reached by the use of this knowledge. Equipped with this book alone, one could perform seeming miracles in changing the states of health, ability and intelligence of people. This *is* how life works. This *is* how you change men, women and children for the better, and attain greater personal freedom.

A New Slant on Life • Have you ever asked yourself Who am I? What am I? This book of articles by L. Ron Hubbard answers these all-too-common questions. This is knowledge one can use every day—for a new, more confident and happier slant on life!

The Problems of Work • Work plays a big part in the game of life. Do you really enjoy your work? Are you certain of your job security? Would you like the increased personal satisfaction of doing your work well? This is the book that shows exactly how to achieve these things and more. The game of life—and within it, the game of work—can be enjoyable and rewarding.

Scientology 0-8: The Book of Basics • What is life? Did you know an individual can create space, energy and time? Here are the basics of life itself, and the secrets of becoming cause over any area of your life. Discover how you can use the data in this book to achieve your goals.

Basic Dictionary of Dianetics and Scientology • Compiled from the works of L. Ron Hubbard, this convenient dictionary contains the terms and expressions needed by anyone learning Dianetics and Scientology technology. And a *special bonus*—an easy-to-read Scientology organizing board chart that shows you who to contact for services and information at your nearest Scientology organization.

Basic Dianetics Books

The Basic Dianetics Books Package is your complete guide to the inner workings of the mind. You can get all of these books individually or in a set, complete with an attractive slipcase.

Dianetics: The Modern Science of Mental Health • Acclaimed as the most effective self-help book ever published. Dianetics technology has helped millions reach new heights of freedom and ability. Millions of copies are sold every year! Discover the source of mental barriers that prevent you from achieving your goals—and how to handle them!

The Dynamics of Life • Break through the barriers to your happiness. This is the first book Ron wrote detailing the startling principles behind Dianetics—facts so powerful they can change forever the way you look at yourself and your potentials. Discover how you can use the powerful basic principles in this book to blast through the barriers of your mind and gain full control over your success, future and happiness.

Self Analysis • The complete do-it-yourself handbook for anyone who wants to improve their abilities and success potential. Use the simple, easy-to-learn techniques in *Self Analysis* to build self-confidence and reduce stress.

Dianetics: The Evolution of a Science • It is estimated that we use less than 10 percent of our mind's potential. What stops us from developing and using the full potential of our minds? *Dianetics: The Evolution of a Science* is L. Ron Hubbard's incredible story of how he discovered the reactive mind and how he developed the keys to unlock its secrets. Get this firsthand account of what the mind really is, and how you can release its hidden potential.

Dianetics Graduate Books

These books by L. Ron Hubbard give you detailed knowledge of how the mind works—data you can use to help yourself and others break out of the traps of life. While you can get these books individually, the Dianetics Graduate Books Package can also be purchased as a set, complete with an attractive slipcase.

Science of Survival • If you ever wondered why people act the way they do, you'll find this book a wealth of information. It's vital to anyone who wants to understand others and improve personal relationships. *Science of Survival* is built around a remarkable chart—The Hubbard Chart of Human Evaluation. With it you can understand and predict other people's behavior and reactions and greatly increase your control over your own life. This is a valuable handbook that can make a difference between success and failure on the job and in life.

Dianetics 55! • Your success in life depends on your ability to communicate. Do you know a formula exists for communication? Learn the rules of better communication that can help you live a more fulfilling life. Here, L. Ron Hubbard deals with the fundamental principles of communication and how you can master these to achieve your goals.

Advanced Procedure and Axioms • For the *first* time the basics of thought and the physical universe have been codified into a set of fundamental laws, signaling an entirely new way to view and approach the subjects of man, the physical universe and even life itself.

Handbook for Preclears • Written as an advanced personal workbook, *Handbook for Preclears* contains easily done processes to help you overcome the effect of times you were not in control of your life, times that your emotions were a barrier to your success and much more. Completing all the fifteen auditing steps contained in this book sets you up for really being in *control* of your environment and life.

Child Dianetics • Here is a revolutionary new approach to rearing children with Dianetics auditing techniques. Find out how you can help your child achieve greater confidence, more self-reliance, improved learning rate and a happier, more loving relationship with you.

Notes on the Lectures of L. Ron Hubbard • Compiled from his fascinating lectures given shortly after the publication of *Dianetics*, this book contains some of the first material Ron ever released on the ARC Triangle and the Tone Scale, and how these discoveries relate to auditing.

OT[1] Library Package

All the following books contain the knowledge of a spiritual being's relationship to this universe and how his abilities to operate successfully in it can be restored. You can get all of

---

1. **OT:** abbreviation for **Operating Thetan,** a state of beingness. It is a being "at cause over matter, energy, space, time, form and life." *Operating* comes from "able to operate without dependency on things," and *thetan* is the Greek letter *theta* (θ) which the Greeks used to represent *thought* or perhaps *spirit*, to which an *n* is added to make a noun in the modern style used to create words in engineering. It is also θ^n or "theta to the nth degree," meaning unlimited or vast.

these books individually or in a set, complete with an attractive slipcase.

Scientology 8-80 • What are the laws of life? We are all familiar with physical laws such as the law of gravity, but what laws govern life and thought? L. Ron Hubbard answers the riddles of life and its goals in the physical universe.

Scientology 8-8008 • Get the basic truths about your nature as a spiritual being and your relationship to the physical universe around you. Here, L. Ron Hubbard describes procedures designed to increase your abilities to heights previously only dreamed of.

Scientology: A History of Man • A fascinating look at the evolutionary background and history of the human race— revolutionary concepts guaranteed to intrigue you and challenge many basic assumptions about man's true power, potential and abilities.

The Creation of Human Ability • This book contains processes designed to restore the power of a thetan over his own postulates, to understand the nature of his beingness, to free his self-determinism and much, much more.

Basic Executive Books

The Basic Executive Books Package consists of the book *Problems of Work* and the two books listed below. They are available individually or as a set, complete with an attractive slipcase.

How to Live Though an Executive • What are the factors in business and commerce which, if lacking, can keep a person overworked and worried, keep labor and management at each other's throats, and make an unsafe working atmosphere? L. Ron Hubbard reveals principles based on years of research into many different types of organizations.

Introduction to Scientology Ethics • A complete knowledge of ethics is vital to anyone's success in life. Without knowing and applying the information in this book, success is only a matter of luck or chance. That is not much to look forward to. This book contains the answers to questions like, "How do I know when a decision is right or wrong?" "How can I predictably improve things around me?" The powerful ethics technology of L. Ron Hubbard is your way to ever-increasing survival.

Other Scientology Books

Have You Lived Before This Life? • This is the book that sparked a flood of interest in the ancient puzzle: Does man live only one life? The answer lay in mystery, buried until L. Ron Hubbard's researches unearthed the truth. Actual case histories of people recalling past lives in auditing tell the tale.

Dianetics and Scientology Technical Dictionary • This dictionary is your indispensable guide to the words and ideas of Scientology and Dianetics technologies—technologies which can help you increase your know-how and effectiveness in life. Over three thousand words are defined—including a new understanding of vital words like *life, love* and *happiness* as well as Scientology terms.

Modern Management Technology Defined: Hubbard Dictionary of Administration and Management • Here's a real breakthrough in the subject of administration and management! Eighty-six hundred words are defined for greater understanding of any business situation. Clear, precise Scientology definitions describe many previously baffling phenomena and bring truth, sanity and understanding to the often murky field of business management.

Organization Executive Course • The *Organization Executive Course* volumes contain organizational technology never before known to man. This is not just how a Scientology organization works; this is how the operation of *any* organization, *any* activity, can be improved. A person knowing the data in these volumes fully, and applying it, could completely reverse any downtrend in a company—or even a country!

Management Series Volumes 1 and 2 • These books contain technology that anyone who works with management in any way must know completely to be a true success. Contained in these books are such subjects as data evaluation, the technology of how to organize any area for maximum production and expansion, how to handle personnel, the actual technology of public relations and much more.

Background and Ceremonies of the Church of Scientology • Discover the beautiful and inspiring ceremonies of the Church of Scientology, and its fascinating religious and historical background. This book contains the illuminating Creed of the Church, church services, sermons and ceremonies, many as originally given in person by L. Ron Hubbard, Founder of Scientology.

What Is Scientology? • Scientology philosophy has attracted great interest and attention since its beginning. What is Scientology philosophy? What can it accomplish—and why are so many people from all walks of life proclaiming its effectiveness? Find the answers to these questions and many others in *What Is Scientology?*

Introductory and Demonstration Processes and Assists • How can you help someone increase his enthusiasm for living? How can you improve someone's self-confidence on the job? Here are basic Scientology processes you can use to help others deal with life and living.

Volunteer Minister's Handbook • This is a big, practical how-to-do-it book to give a person the basic knowledge on how to help self and others through the rough spots in life. It consists of twenty-one sections—each one covering important situations in life, such as drug and alcohol problems, study difficulties, broken marriages, accidents and illnesses, a failing business, difficult children, and much more. This is the basic tool you need to help someone out of troubles, and bring about a happier life.

The Personal Achievement Series

There are nearly three thousand recorded lectures by L. Ron Hubbard on the subjects of Dianetics and Scientology. What follows is a sampling of these lectures, each known and loved the world over. All of these are presented in CLEARSOUND™ state-of-the-art sound-recording technology, notable for its clarity and brilliance of reproduction.

Get all the Personal Achievement Series cassettes by L. Ron Hubbard listed below and ask your nearest Scientology church or organization or the publisher about future releases.

The Story of Dianetics and Scientology • In this lecture, L. Ron Hubbard shares with you his earliest insights into human nature and gives a compelling and often humorous account of his experiences. Spend an unforgettable time with Ron as he talks about the start of Dianetics and Scientology!

The Road to Truth • The road to truth has eluded man since the beginning of time. In this classic lecture, L. Ron Hubbard explains what this road actually is and why it is the only road one MUST travel all the way once begun. This lecture reveals the only road to higher levels of living.

Scientology and Effective Knowledge • Voyage to new horizons of awareness! *Scientology and Effective Knowledge* by

L. Ron Hubbard can help you understand more about yourself and others. A fascinating tale of the beginnings of Dianetics and Scientology.

The Deterioration of Liberty • What do governments fear so much in a population that they amass weapons to defend themselves from people? Find out from Ron in this classic lecture.

Power of Choice and Self-Determinism • Man's ability to determine the course of his life depends on his ability to exercise his power of choice. Find how you can increase your power of choice and self-determinism in life from Ron in this lecture.

Scientology and Ability • Ron points out that this universe is here because we perceive it and agree to it. Applying Scientology principles to life can bring new adventure to life and put you on the road to discovering better beingness.

The Hope of Man • Various men in history brought forth the idea that there was hope of improvement. But L. Ron Hubbard's discoveries in Dianetics and Scientology have made that hope a reality. Find out by listening to this lecture how Scientology has become man's one, true hope for his final freedom.

The Dynamics • In this lecture Ron gives incredible data on the dynamics: how man creates on them; what happens when a person gets stuck in just one; how wars relate to the third dynamic and much more.

Money • Ron talks in this classic lecture about that subject which makes or breaks men with the greatest of ease—money. Find out what money really is and gain greater control over your own finances.

Formulas for Success—*The Five Conditions* • How does one achieve real success? It sometimes appears that luck is the primary factor, but the truth of the matter is that natural laws exist which govern the conditions of life. These laws have been discovered by Ron, and in this lecture he gives you the exact steps to take in order to improve conditions in any aspect of your life.

Health and Certainty • You need certainty of yourself in order to achieve the success you want in life. In *Health and Certainty*, L. Ron Hubbard tells how you can achieve certainty and really be free to think for yourself. Get this tape now and start achieving your full potential!

Operation Manual for the Mind • Everybody has a mind— but who has an operation manual for it? This lecture reveals why man went on for thousands of years without understanding how his mind is supposed to work. The problem has been solved. Find out how with this tape.

Miracles • Why is it that man often loses to those forces he resists or opposes? Why can't an individual simply overcome obstacles in life and win? In the tape lecture *Miracles*, L. Ron Hubbard describes why one suffers losses in life. He also describes how a person can experience the miracles of happiness, self-fulfillment and winning at life. Get a copy today.

The Road to Perfection—*The Goodness of Man* • Unlike earlier practices that sought to "improve" man because he was "bad," Scientology assumes that you have *good* qualities that simply need to be *increased*. In *The Road to Perfection*, L. Ron Hubbard shows how workable this assumption really is—and how you can begin to use your mind, talents and abilities to the fullest. Get this lecture and increase your ability to handle life.

The Dynamic Principles of Existence • What does it take to survive in today's world? It's not something you learn much about in school. You have probably gotten a lot of advice about how to "get along." *Your survival right now is limited by the data you were given.* This lecture describes the dynamic principles of existence, and tells how you can use these principles to increase your success in all areas of life. Happiness and self-esteem *can* be yours. Don't settle for anything less.

Man: Good or Evil? • In this lecture, L. Ron Hubbard explores the greatest mystery that has confronted modern science and philosophy—the true nature of man's livingness and beingness. Is man simply a sort of wind-up doll or clock—or worse, an evil beast with no control of his cravings? Or is he capable of reaching higher levels of ability, awareness and happiness? Get this tape and find out the *real* answers.

Differences between Scientology and Other Studies • The most important questions in life are the ones you started asking as a child: What happens to a person when he dies? Is man basically good, or is he evil? What are the intentions of the world toward me? Did my mother and father really love me? What is love? Unlike other studies, which try to *force* you to think a certain way, Scientology enables you to find your own answers. Listen to this important lecture. It will put you on the road to true understanding and belief in yourself.

The Machinery of the Mind • We do a lot of things "automatically"—such as driving a car. But what happens when a person's mental machinery takes over and starts running him? In this fascinating lecture, L. Ron Hubbard gives you an understanding of what mental machinery really is, and how it can cause a person to lose control. You *can* regain your power of decision and be in full control of your life. Listen to this lecture and find out how.

The Affinity–Reality–Communication Triangle • Have you ever tried to talk to an angry man? Have you ever tried to get something across to someone who is really in fear? Have you ever known someone who was impossible to cheer up? Listen to this fascinating lecture by L. Ron Hubbard and learn how you can use the affinity-reality-communication triangle to resolve personal relationships. By using the data in this lecture, you can better understand others and live a happier life.

Increasing Efficiency • Inefficiency is a major barrier to success. How can you increase your efficiency? Is it a matter of changing your diet, or adjusting your working environment? These approaches have uniformly failed, because they overlook the most important element: *you*. L. Ron Hubbard has found those factors that *can* increase your efficiency, and he reveals it in this timely lecture. Get *Increasing Efficiency* now, and start achieving *your* full potential.

Man's Relentless Search • For countless centuries, man has been trying to find himself. Why does this quest repeatedly end in frustration and disappointment? What is he *really* looking for, and why can't he find it? For the real truth about man and life, listen to this taped lecture by L. Ron Hubbard, *Man's Relentless Search*. Restore your belief in yourself!

More advanced books and lectures are available. Contact your nearest organization or write directly to the publisher for a full catalog.

Get Your Free Catalog of Knowledge on How to Improve Life

L. Ron Hubbard's books and tapes increase your ability to understand yourself and others. His works give you the practical know-how you need to improve your life and the lives of your family and friends.

Many more materials by L. Ron Hubbard are available than have been covered in the pages of this book. A free catalog of these materials is available on request.

Write for your free catalog today!

Bridge Publications, Inc.
4751 Fountain Avenue
Los Angeles, California 90029

NEW ERA Publications International, ApS
Store Kongensgade 55
1264 Copenhagen K, Denmark

"I am always happy to hear from my readers."

L. Ron Hubbard

These were the words of L. Ron Hubbard, who was always very interested in hearing from his friends and readers. He made a point of staying in communication with everyone he came in contact with over his fifty-year career as a professional writer, and he had thousands of fans and friends that he corresponded with all over the world.

The publishers of L. Ron Hubbard's works wish to continue this tradition and welcome letters and comments from you, his readers, both old and new.

Additionally, the publishers will be happy to send you information on anything you would like to know about Ron, his extraordinary life and accomplishments and the vast number of books he has written.

Any message addressed to the Author's Affairs Director at Bridge Publications will be given prompt and full attention.

Bridge Publications, Inc.
4751 Fountain Avenue
Los Angeles, California 90029
USA

Church and Organization Address List

United States of America

Albuquerque
Church of Scientology
8106 Menaul Blvd. NE
Albuquerque, New Mexico 87110

Ann Arbor
Church of Scientology
301 North Ingalls Street
Ann Arbor, Michigan 48104

Atlanta
Church of Scientology
2632 Piedmonte Rd., NE
Atlanta, Georgia 30324

Austin
Church of Scientology
2200 Guadalupe
Austin, Texas 78705

Boston
Church of Scientology
448 Beacon Street
Boston, Massachusetts 02115

Buffalo
Church of Scientology
47 West Huron Street
Buffalo, New York 14202

Chicago
Church of Scientology
3011 North Lincoln Avenue
Chicago, Illinois 60657

Cincinnati
Church of Scientology
215 West 4th Street, 5th Floor
Cincinnati, Ohio 45202

Clearwater
Church of Scientology
Flag® Service Organization
210 South Fort Harrison Avenue
Clearwater, Florida 34616

Columbus
Church of Scientology
167 East State Street
Columbus, Ohio 43215

Dallas
Church of Scientology
Celebrity Centre® Dallas
8501 Manderville Lane
Dallas, Texas 75231

Denver
Church of Scientology
375 South Navajo Street
Denver, Colorado 80223

Detroit
Church of Scientology
321 Williams Street
Royal Oak, Michigan 48067

Honolulu
Church of Scientology
1 N. King St., Lower Level
Honolulu, Hawaii 96817

Kansas City
Church of Scientology
3619 Broadway
Kansas City, Missouri 64111

Las Vegas
Church of Scientology
846 East Sahara Avenue
Las Vegas, Nevada 89104

Church of Scientology
Celebrity Centre Las Vegas
1100 South 10th Street
Las Vegas, Nevada 89104-1505

Long Island
Church of Scientology
330 Fulton Avenue
Hempstead, New York 11550

Los Angeles and vicinity
Church of Scientology
4810 Sunset Boulevard
Los Angeles, California 90027

Church of Scientology
1451 Irvine Boulevard
Tustin, California 92680

Church of Scientology
99 East Colorado Boulevard
Pasadena, California 91150

Church of Scientology
10335 Magnolia Boulevard
North Hollywood, California 91601

Church of Scientology
American Saint Hill Organization
1413 North Berendo Street
Los Angeles, California 90027

Church of Scientology
American Saint Hill Foundation
1413 North Berendo Street
Los Angeles, California 90027

Church of Scientology
Advanced Organization of
   Los Angeles
1306 North Berendo Street
Los Angeles, California 90027

Church of Scientology
Celebrity Centre International
5930 Franklin Avenue
Hollywood, California 90028

Miami
Church of Scientology
120 Giralda Avenue
Coral Gables, Florida 33134

Minneapolis
Church of Scientology
3019 Minnehaha Avenue
Minneapolis, Minnesota 55406

New Haven
Church of Scientology
909 Whalley Avenue
New Haven, Connecticut 06515

New York City
Church of Scientology
227 West 46th Street
New York City, New York 10036

Church of Scientology
Celebrity Centre New York
65 East 82nd Street
New York City, New York 10028

Orlando
Church of Scientology
710-A East Colonial Drive
Orlando, Florida 32803

Philadelphia
Church of Scientology
1315 Race Street
Philadelphia, Pennsylvania 19107

Phoenix
Church of Scientology
4450 North Central Avenue, Suite 102
Phoenix, Arizona 85012

Portland
Church of Scientology
323 SW Washington
Portland, Oregon 97204

Church of Scientology
Celebrity Centre Portland
709 Southwest Salmon Street
Portland, Oregon 97205

Sacramento
Church of Scientology
825 15th Street
Sacramento, California 95814

San Diego
Church of Scientology
701 "C" Street
San Diego, California 92101

San Francisco
Church of Scientology
83 McAllister Street
San Francisco, California 94102

San Jose
Church of Scientology
80 E. Rosemary
San Jose, California 95112

Santa Barbara
Church of Scientology
524 State Street
Santa Barbara, California 93101

Seattle
Church of Scientology
2004 Westlake Avenue
Seattle, Washington 98121

St. Louis
Church of Scientology
9510 Page Boulevard
St. Louis, Missouri 63132

Tampa
Church of Scientology
4809 North Armenia Avenue
Suite 215
Tampa, Florida 33603

Washington, DC
Founding Church of Scientology
2125 "S" Street NW
Washington, DC 20008

Canada

Edmonton
Church of Scientology
10349 82nd Avenue
Edmonton, Alberta
Canada T6E 1Z9

Kitchener
Church of Scientology
8 Water Street North
Kitchener, Ontario
Canada N2H 5A5

Montréal
Church of Scientology
4489 Papineau Street
Montréal, Québec
Canada H2H 1T7

Ottawa
Church of Scientology
150 Rideau Street, 2nd Floor
Ottawa, Ontario
Canada K1N 5X6

Quèbec
Church of Scientology
226 St-Joseph est
Québec, Québec
Canada G1K 3A9

Toronto
Church of Scientology
696 Yonge Street
Toronto, Ontario
Canada M4Y 2A7

Vancouver
Church of Scientology
401 West Hastings Street
Vancouver, British Columbia
Canada V6B 1L5

Winnipeg
Church of Scientology
Suite 125—388 Donald Street
Winnipeg, Manitoba
Canada R3B 2J4

United Kingdom

Birmingham
Church of Scientology
60/62 Constitution Hill
Birmingham
England B19 3JT

Brighton
Church of Scientology
Dukes Arcade, Top Floor
Dukes Street
Brighton, Sussex
England

East Grinstead
Saint Hill Foundation
Saint Hill Manor
East Grinstead, West Sussex
England RH19 4JY

Advanced Organization Saint Hill
Saint Hill Manor
East Grinstead, West Sussex
England RH19 4JY

Edinburgh

Hubbard Academy of Personal
    Independence
20 Southbridge
Edinburgh, Scotland EH1 1LL

London

Church of Scientology
68 Tottenham Court Road
London, England W1P 0BB

Manchester

Church of Scientology
258 Deansgate
Manchester, England M3 4BG

Plymouth

Church of Scientology
41 Ebrington Street
Plymouth, Devon
England PL4 9AA

Sunderland

Church of Scientology
51 Fawcett Street
Sunderland, Tyne and Wear
England SR1 1RS

Austria

Vienna

Church of Scientology
Schottenfeldgasse 13–15
1070 Vienna, Austria

Vienna South

Church of Scientology
Celebrity Centre VNA
Senefelderg. 12
A-1100 Vienna, Austria

Belgium

Brussels

Church of Scientology
45A, rue de l'Ecuyer
1000 Bruxelles, Belgium

Denmark

Aarhus

Church of Scientology
Guldsmedegade 17, 2
8000 Aarhus C, Denmark

Copenhagen

Church of Scientology
Store Kongensgade 55
1264 Copenhagen K, Denmark

Church of Scientology
Vesterbrogade 66
1620 Copenhagen V, Denmark

Church of Scientology
Advanced Organization Saint Hill
    for Europe and Africa
Jernbanegade 6
1608 Copenhagen V, Denmark

France

Angers

Church of Scientology
10–12, rue Max Richard
49000 Angers, France

Clermont-Ferrand

Church of Scientology
2 Pte rue Giscard de la Tour Fondue
63000 Clermont-Ferrand, France

Lyon

Church of Scientology
3, place des Capucins
69001 Lyon, France

Paris

Church of Scientology
65, rue de Dunkerque
75009 Paris, France

Church of Scientology
Celebrity Centre Paris
69, rue Legendre
75017 Paris, France

St. Etienne

Church of Scientology
24, rue Marengo
42000 St. Etienne, France

Germany

Berlin
Church of Scientology e.V.
Sponholzstrasse 51/52
1000 Berlin 41, Germany

Düsseldorf
Church of Scientology
Friedrichstrasse 28
4000 Düsseldorf, West Germany

Church of Scientology
Celebrity Centre Düsseldorf
Grupellostr. 28
4000 Düsseldorf, West Germany

Frankfurt
Church of Scientology
Darmstadter Landstrasse 213
6000 Frankfurt 70, West Germany

Hamburg
Church of Scientology e.V.
Steindamm 63
2000 Hamburg 1, West Germany

Church of Scientology
Celebrity Centre Hamburg
Mönckebergstrasse 5/IV
2000 Hamburg 1
West Germany

Hanover
Church of Scientology
Hubertusstrasse 2
D-3000 Hannover 1, West Germany

Munich
Church of Scientology e.V.
Beichstrasse 12
D-8000 München 40, West Germany

Stuttgart
Church of Scientology
Hirschstrasse 27
7000 Stuttgart, West Germany

Greece

Athens
Applied Philosophy Center of Greece
  (K.E.F.E.)
Ippokratous 175B
114 72 Athens, Greece

Israel

Tel Aviv
Scientology and Dianetics College
7 Salomon Street
Tel Aviv 66023, Israel

Italy

Brescia
Church of Scientology
Dei Tre Laghi
Via Fratelli Bronzetti N. 20
25125 Brescia, Italy

Milano
Church of Scientology
Via Abetone, 10
20137 Milano, Italy

Monza
Church of Scientology
Via Cavour, 5
20052 Monza, Italy

Novara
Church of Scientology
Corso Cavallotti No. 7
28100 Novara, Italy

Nuoro
Church of Scientology
Via G. Deledda, 43
08100 Nuoro, Italy

Padua
Church of Scientology
Via Mameli 1/5
35131 Padova, Italy

Pordenone
Church of Scientology
Via Montereale, 10/C
33170 Pordenone, Italy

Rome
Church of Scientology
Via di San Vito, 11
00185 Roma, Italy

Turin
Church of Scientology
Via Guarini, 4
10121 Torino, Italy

Verona
Church of Scientology
Vicolo Chiodo No. 4/A
37121 Verona, Italy

Netherlands

Amsterdam
Church of Scientology
Nieuwe Zijds Voorburgwal 271
1012 RL Amsterdam, Netherlands

Norway

Oslo
Church of Scientology
Storgata 9
0155 Oslo 1, Norway

Portugal

Lisbon
Instituto de Dianética
Rua Actor Taborda 39–4°
1000 Lisboa, Portugal

Spain

Barcelona
Dianética
Calle Pau Claris 85, Principal 1ª
08010 Barcelona, Spain

Madrid
Asociación Civil de Dianética
Montera 20, Piso 1° DCHA
28013 Madrid, Spain

Sweden

Göteborg
Church of Scientology
Odinsgatan 8
411 03 Göteborg, Sweden

Malmö
Church of Scientology
Simrishamnsgatan 10
21423 Malmö, Sweden

Stockholm
Church of Scientology
Kammakargatan 46
S-111 60 Stockholm, Sweden

Switzerland

Basel
Church of Scientology
Herrengrabenweg 56
4054 Basel, Switzerland

Bern
Church of Scientology
Schulhausgasse 12
3113 Rubigen
Bern, Switzerland

Geneva
Church of Scientology
9 Route de Saint-Julien
1227 Carouge
Genève, Switzerland

Lausanne
Church of Scientology
10, rue de la Madeleine
1003 Lausanne, Switzerland

Zürich
Church of Scientology
Badenerstrasse 294
CH-8004 Zürich, Switzerland

Australia

Adelaide
Church of Scientology
24 Waymouth Street
Adelaide, South Australia 5000
Australia

Brisbane
Church of Scientology
2nd Floor, 106 Edward Street
Brisbane, Queensland 4000
Australia

Canberra
Church of Scientology
Suite 16, 108 Bunda Street
Canberra Civic
A.C.T. 2601, Australia

Melbourne
Church of Scientology
44 Russell Street
Melbourne, Victoria 3000
Australia

Perth
Church of Scientology
39–41 King Street
Perth, Western Australia 6000
Australia

Sydney
Church of Scientology
201 Castlereagh Street
Sydney, New South Wales 2000
Australia

Church of Scientology
Advanced Organization Saint Hill
  Australia, New Zealand and
  Oceania
19–37 Greek Street
Glebe, New South Wales 2037
Australia

Japan

Tokyo
Scientology Organization
101 Toyomi Nishi Gotanda Heights
2-13-5 Nishi Gotanda
Shinagawa-Ku
Tokyo, Japan 141

New Zealand

Auckland
Church of Scientology
32 Lorne Street
Auckland 1, New Zealand

Africa

Bulawayo
Church of Scientology
74 Abercorn Street
Bulawayo, Zimbabwe

Cape Town
Church of Scientology
5 Beckham Street
Gardens
Cape Town 8001, South Africa

Durban
Church of Scientology
57 College Lane
Durban 4001, South Africa

Harare
Church of Scientology
First Floor State Lottery Building
P.O. Box 3524
Corner Speke Avenue and
  Julius Nyerere Way
Harare, Zimbabwe

Johannesburg
Church of Scientology
Security Building, 2nd Floor
95 Commissioner Street
Johannesburg 2001, South Africa

Church of Scientology
101 Huntford Building
40 Hunter Street
Cnr. Hunter & Fortesque Roads
Yeoville 2198
Johannesburg, South Africa

Port Elizabeth
Church of Scientology
2 St. Christopher
27 Westbourne Road
  Central
Port Elizabeth 6001, South Africa

Pretoria
Church of Scientology
1st Floor City Centre
272 Pretorius Street
Pretoria 0002, South Africa

Latin America

Colombia

Bogotá
Centro Cultural de Dianética
Carrera 19 No. 39–55
Apartado Aereo 92419
Bogotá, D.E. Colombia

Mexico

Estado de México
Instituto Technologico de Dianética,
  A.C.
Londres 38, 5th Floor
Col. Juarez, México D.F.

Guadalajara
Organización Cultural Dianética de
  Guadalajara, A.C.
Av. Lopez Mateos Nte. 329
Sector Hidalgo
Guadalajara, Jalisco, México

Mexico City

Asociación Cultural Dianética, A.C.
Hermes No. 46
Colonia Crédito Constructor
03940 México 19, D.F.

Instituto de Filosofia Aplicada, A.C.
Durango #105
Colonia Roma
06700 México D.F.

Instituto de Filosofia Aplicada, A.C.
Plaza Rio de Janeiro No. 52
Colonia Roma
06700 México D.F.

Organización, Desarrollo y
    Dianética, A.C.
Providencia 1000
Colonia Del Valle
C.P. 03100 México D.F.

Centro de Dianética Polanco
Insurgentes Sur 536, 1er piso
    Esq. Nogales
Colonia Roma Sur C.P.
06700 México D.F.

Venezuela

Valencia

Asociación Cultural Dianética de
    Venezuela, A.C.
Ave. 101 No. 150–23
Urbanizacion La Alegria
Apartado Postal 833
Valencia, Venezuela

To obtain any books or cassettes by L. Ron Hubbard which are not available at your local organization, contact any of the following publishers:

Bridge Publications, Inc.
4751 Fountain Avenue
Los Angeles, California 90029

Continental Publications Liaison
Office
696 Yonge Street
Toronto, Ontario
Canada M4Y 2A7

NEW ERA Publications International,
    ApS
Store Kongensgade 55
1264 Copenhagen K, Denmark

Era Dinámica Editores, S.A. de C.V.
Alabama 105
Colonia Nápoles
C.P. 03810 México, D.F.

NEW ERA Publications, Ltd.
78 Holmethorpe Avenue
Redhill, Surrey RH1 2NL
United Kingdom

N.E. Publications Australia Pty. Ltd.
2 Verona Street
Paddington, New South Wales 2021
Australia

Continental Publications Pty. Ltd.
P.O. Box 27080
Benrose 2011
South Africa

NEW ERA Publications Italia Srl
Via L.G. Columella, 12
20128 Milano, Italy

NEW ERA Publications GmbH
Otto—Hahn—Strasse 25
6072 Dreieich 1, Germany

NEW ERA Publications France
111, Boulevard de Magenta
75010 Paris, France

New Era Publications España, S.A.
C/De la Paz, 4/1° dcha
28012 Madrid, Spain

New Era Japan
5-4-5-803 Nishigotanda
Shinagawa-Ku
Tokyo, Japan 141